GLYPHOSATE FREE

An essay on
functional nutrition
and the
homeopathic clearing
of glyphosate toxicity

Kate Birch, RSHom(NA), CCH

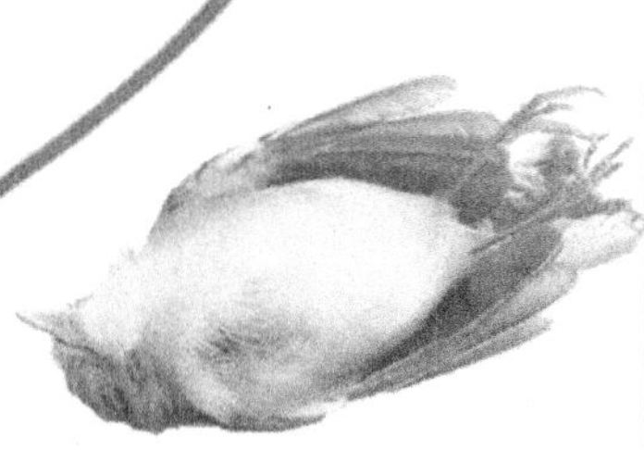

Interior Design and Layout: Kate Birch

Cover design: Kate Birch. Images are sourced from the internet.

Editing: Chrissy Moore, Anna Gray, Sarah Damlo

ISBN-13: 9781721930678

ISBN-10: 1721930671

Printed in the United States of America

Publication date: 3/3/2019

Dedication

For Humanity and the Earth

This is a call to realize that we are of nature. Our actions towards nature have direct ramifications in our lives.

This is a call to humanity to search for truth in our incarnation and participation in this earthly existence.

We are here to protect the planet and its inhabitants.

This earth gives us the air we breathe, the water we drink, grows the food that feeds us, and the trees we use to build our homes.

It is time we stop violating and polluting the earth because of our feelings of lack.

This feeling of lack leads us to think we need toxic chemicals and genetically modified crops to feed us.

This illness is going to destroy the genetic code of our Creation and the biome of the earth. It will kill us all.

For the sake of every living being's salvation and survival on this planet it is time we have respect for, trust in, and work with, the abundance of nature to provide for our needs.

May all beings be healthy.

Other Books by Kate Birch

- **Vaccine Free Prevention and Treatment of Infectious Contagious Disease with Homeopathy**

- **Homeopathic Therapeutics of the Liver and Biliary Ducts ~ The Amazing Liver: Interfacing Nature with Spirit**

- **The Best Family Homeopathy Acute Care Manual**

Co-author of

- **The Solution ~ Homeoprophylaxis: The Vaccine Alternative**

Acknowledgements

If it were not for the dedicated researchers and scientists who have spent their life's work exposing the toxicity of glyphosate this essay would not have been possible.

Here I would like to thank specifically Stephanie Seneff and Judy Mikovits, both of whom I have met several times at national conferences and public platforms. Their contributions to the revelatory science and truth behind glyphosate, DNA, biome and vaccines has been exemplary.

I would like to thank all the other researchers from around the world for their part in the study of glyphosate.

I would like to thank my clients who have been my teachers, and ultimately the ability of my psyche to work through my own personal difficulties in accepting the facts as I have presented them here for you.

Thank you, to my editing and review team Chrissy Moore, Kristen Linner PhD, Anna Gray, and Sarah Damlo. Your input has been invaluable.

Cover Art: *By design humans, and all living beings and their sacred DNA, are in perfect order. The blueprint of Creation is depicted by the DNA strand on the back cover. On the front, the radiant sun beams its light from behind the Golden Ratio. The sun is the earth's healer and vital force generator that gives all plants life. Juxtaposed is the shadow over the sun, obscuring it, reflective of the pollution fracturing its pure light. The image of a crop duster spraying GMO crops is active pollution of the planet and our food sources. The dead canary on the title page symbolizes the struggles of those who are the first to succumb to the poisoning. May we take heed to the canary and free ourselves from our own demise.*

The Golden Ratio: *A depiction of the perfection found in nature and in the essential Man. It is Man's duty to bring his comprehension and actions in line with the perfection of his essence. The use of glyphosate and genetic modification of foods, and resultant limitations in human, animal and plant epigenetics, is not only an act against nature but an act against all living beings.*

Foreword

Life is a journey and finding truth is not always an easy path. Throughout my life I was burdened with asthma, acne, and sinus infections. Always taking the conventional medicine route, I was administered inhalers and prescriptions from an early age into adulthood. It was not until I became a mother that I began to question my health, my family's health, and the advice given by the medical establishment.

I was introduced to homeopathy in 2012. I am amazed how the body can heal itself when it is given the right remedy and the organs can perform their rightful duties as they were designed. Lifestyle, nutrition, and homeopathy are key to a healthy life. What is upsetting our health equation are the toxins that our bodies are introduced to and we must try to overcome them in order to maintain health.

My father was diagnosed with lymphatic leukemia three years ago. For the past 15 years he farmed soybeans and sprayed Roundup on these "Roundup-Ready" GMO crops. Living in South Carolina, the dead trees and weeds underneath the power lines are visible signs that they have been sprayed with weed killer. Residential ditches are lined with dead grass after routinely being sprayed to maintain order. The chemical makes its way into our creeks, rivers, lakes, oceans, our ground water and ultimately, in the food and water that we consume. Our world is being inundated with chemicals.

It is vital to find a solution to this endless spraying that is causing havoc to our environment and in our bodies. Getting back to the basics is essential. Ridding our bodies of this toxic chemical and living a healthy lifestyle ensures that future generations have that opportunity. Finding truth and living a life that is in constant pursuit of truth is important.

Throughout the process of editing this book I have been learning about the chemical glyphosate and the subsequent damage that occurs when introduced to the human body. I am learning how to detox and restore health after being impacted by this toxin. Striving for optimal health is the goal. I have been assisting my father, for the past two years to integrate healthy nutrition, different forms of detox, and homeopathy to help support his system. Dealing with glyphosate is "new" and unchartered territory. The journey of learning and incorporating change is tedious but necessary to reestablish one's health.

Like myself, Kate Birch believes that homeopathy provides the clearest roadmap to a healthy, holistic way of living to fulfill the health equation.

Kate Birch is a homeopathic professional with over 24 years of clinical practice. She has been administering homeopathic advice and remedies for me and my family for five years. She is devoted to providing a holistic approach to illness and has been instrumental in teaching and guiding my family to a higher level of health. She is committed to research and finding the right answers. This book is a tool for all who have been touched by the chemical glyphosate. It is rich in instruction for those who want to regain and maintain health while living in a world filled with toxins.

Chrissy Moore,

South Carolina, January 30, 2019.

Preface

Along the way we are exposed to life. We grow, change, experience stress, get sick and if possible, we recover. I never planned on writing a book on glyphosate toxicity until I discovered that I had been poisoned by glyphosate. The reverse was true for my book Vaccine Free Treatment and Prevention of Infectious Contagious Disease with Homeopathy. I never realized that I had vaccine injury until I wrote that book. I was also poisoned with mercury from the amalgam fillings I received when I was a teenager. I do believe the weakness I felt as a youth was partly due to an inherited weakness however, the major confounders in my health was not my inborn weakness but rather the childhood and travel vaccines I had received as a teenager, amalgam toxicity, and glyphosate toxicity.

Fortunately, I came across homeopathy when I was young, and chose to be health conscious regarding the food I ate and the environment I lived in. These choices have restored my health and continues to maintain and improve my health despite living in an ever-toxic world.

How to use this book:

- Review specific sections based on the condition you are studying.
- Reference the index to search for:
  - Symptoms.
  - Diagnosis.
  - Elements and basic building blocks of life.
  - Enzymes, proteins, neurotransmitters, and hormones.
  - Anatomical parts, glands, organs, and organ systems.
  - Nutritional, supplemental, and detox agents.
  - Homeopathic remedies (indicated in bold italic i.e. ***Phosphorus***). *Note: rubrics with remedy abbreviations are not indexed.
- Apply all to the condition you are trying to understand and treat and reference accordingly. For example, when looking at either serotonin imbalance, zonulin, hyperhomocysteinemia, Epstein-Barr virus, or mast cell activation disease, search key words in the index to see all the places they are described, how glyphosate influences, consider the detoxification and nutritional suggestions, and indicated homeopathic remedies.
- Refer to more in-depth homeopathic works for greater understanding of the remedies.

- Seek out a homeopathic practitioner to assist you in your recovery.

This essay is by no means an attempt to diagnose, treat, cure or mitigate any health condition. This essay is an exposé of my journey in the hopes that you may understand how to work with functional nutrition and homeopathy to regain your own health and become glyphosate free. The reader assumes all responsibility for their health outcome from this process. Detox is not just a physical practice. It is a journey into our own salvation.

Through inquiry into the magnitude of the destructive effects of glyphosate toxicity on the foundation of all life, I have simultaneously been inspired by the absolute perfection of the design of the natural world. Whole foods and homeopathic remedies made from the mineral, plant, and animal kingdoms have an innate power to heal. Why, I ask, do humans, as conscious beings, need to push our physical existence to the brink of self-annihilation before we begin to consider how is it we exist in the first place? It is as if the human animal, with his capacity to think, understand, and deduce, has forgotten that he is a part of Creation. We can understand the chemical interactions of the physiological functions in our bodies somehow, yet we have failed to comprehend the effects of our actions towards the very nature that defines us.

While the reader may find themselves falling into a black hole of despair as the outcome seems bleak, I have hope that we will endure, and will change this trajectory. Brace yourself for what is revealed. There is so much more that I have not yet touched upon.

To start with we must work on our individual salvation. It is only by shining the light in the darkness that light prevails. May we all work towards a world where our investment in the planet that houses and feeds us is equal to our investment in our health.

In Service,

Kate Birch, March 1, 2019.

Contents

Open Letter to My State Representative

Dear Sir/Madam,

I am writing to you today to bring to your attention my concern regarding the use of glyphosate in this State (Nation). I personally believe that the entire ecosystem is connected and that a pesticide or herbicide that is sprayed in one location affects the surrounding locations. Glyphosate is the main ingredient in the herbicide and pesticide Roundup. If it can destroy anything living around the crops etc., then it can also work its way up the food chain into all living things.

I personally have experienced glyphosate toxicity and have dealt with a deterioration in my health because of it. Consequently, I choose to buy organic foods and support businesses that do not partake in the use of glyphosate in food production. However, this does not free me from inadvertent exposure such as living down-wind from sprayed crop lands, or from foods that are not labeled correctly. For example, all foods that have soy lecithin in them pose a potential risk, as soybeans are one of the crops most heavily laden with glyphosate. This also harms the bees, amphibians, and wild animals that live within and around the run off from crop lands.

I believe it is the responsibility of our elected officials to oversee regulation of industry according to the cause of environmental justice. All regulation must be targeted to protect people and the environment from harm rather than protecting industry interests.

I also believe that it is the responsibility of our state and federal representative to ensure air and water quality and to implement mandatory water testing for glyphosate in all public water systems and offer free testing for those with private wells, especially those wells in proximity to agricultural lands. Negligence towards these basic needs is negligence towards the electoral constituency you represent.

I am writing to you today to ask you to ensure glyphosate and any other pesticide or herbicide that has the potential to destroy the environment is banned, not only in this State, but on a federal and international level. We want clean air, clean water, and clean food.

In addition, I am asking for the government to support access to organic agriculture. Raw foods, small farmers, and sustainable agricultural practices are the only way to preserve nutritional content of our food, ensure local economies are maintained, and the living beings on this earth thrive.

Next time you have a glass of wine or eat a pizza, know that more than likely it has glyphosate in it unless you have expressly chosen organic or know where it was sourced from. If you or your friends and family suffer from unexplained health conditions, gluten intolerance, thyroid dysfunction, headaches, bloating, cancer, environmental sensitivities, or other conditions, glyphosate may be responsible.

For the sake of my, your, and our children's future, the time to act is now. Toxic agricultural practices are the largest culprit in climate change. It is unknown how much longer life can be supported under these conditions.

Thank you for taking the time to consider these matters and taking appropriate action.

Sincerely,

1. Overview of Glyphosate Exposure

It may seem hard to believe that a substance so ubiquitous could be so harmful to all living organisms on the planet. Unless we do something about this our very survival is at risk. This essay is an introduction to the complications of glyphosate and how to detox it from your body. It is also a plea to find reason and to change what is going on. I want to live my life free of toxins.

There are Four Main Sections in this Essay:

1. Overview of glyphosate and exposure.
2. Basic science of DNA, RNA, and protein structure and the effects of glyphosate on these structures.
3. Symptoms and disease expression of glyphosate toxicity.
4. **How-To** instructions on detoxification of your body with:
    - Nutritional foods and supplements
    - Mechanical detox support
    - Homeopathic treatment and glyphosate clearing
    - Fast and Colon Cleanse

    Woven throughout is the message that we are designed by our creator to be healthy, and if you kill one part of the planet or one aspect of life, it will eventually kill us all. Nature can and will recover from this. Can we?

Glycine or Glyphosate:

Glycine ($C_2H_5NO_2$): is a vitally important, normally occurring, amino acid necessary for a variety of functions within all living organisms. When eating foods that are sprayed with glyphosate, or animals that have eaten crops sprayed with glyphosate, the glyphosate finds its way into all places where the amino acid glycine would normally be used: DNA and RNA transcription, protein and enzyme synthesis, and collagen formation. Glycine serves as an inhibitory neurotransmitter and a precursor to the antioxidant glutathione.

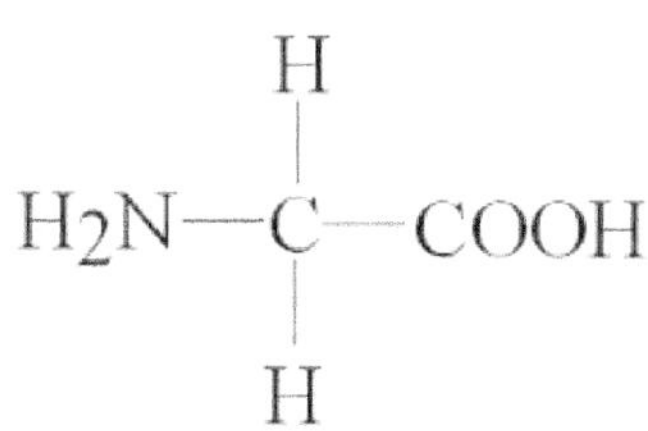

The insertion of glyphosate instead of glycine dysregulates DNA and RNA, which creates junk DNA and RNA that are non-operative, thus disrupts all normal protein synthesis and specific enzyme functionality in all living organisms.[i]

Glyphosate ($C_3H_8NO_5P$): is a water soluble, synthetic substance that is created by joining a glycine molecule with a phosphate molecule. It is a pesticide and herbicide that destroys the enzymatic pathways of bacteria that are a part of the symbiotic process of life and survival. It is found in 'Roundup' and a variety of other commercially available combinations used in different applications on different crops at different times of the year.

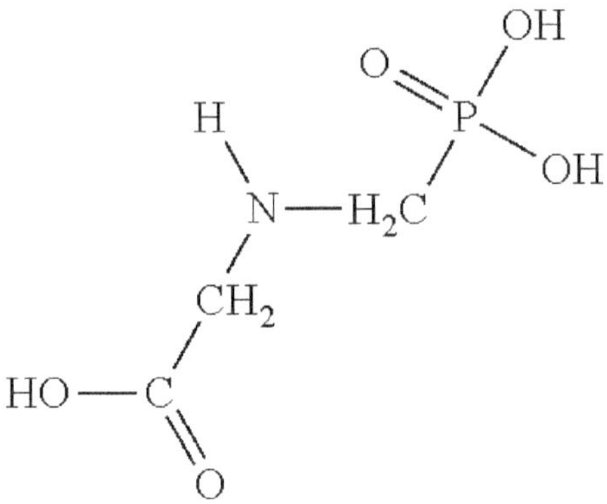

Shikimate-acid Pathway: Glyphosate disrupts the shikimate-acid pathway of bacteria that are present in health and disease in both plants and animals. This pathway is a seven-step metabolic process to make the glycine dependent enzyme 5-enolpyruvylshikimate-3-phosphate (EPSP) synthase. This enzyme is used by beneficial and harmful bacteria, fungi, algae, some protozoan parasites, and in plants for the biosynthesis of folate (B9) and the essential aromatic amino acids (tryptophan, phenylalanine, and tyrosine).

EPSP synthase is produced only by plants and micro-organisms (bacteria); the gene coding for it is not in the mammalian genome. The intestinal flora of some animals makes EPSP synthase (EPSPS). EPSP synthase is the biological target for the pesticide and herbicide glyphosate.

Glyphosate is also a competitive inhibitor of the high energy phosphate ester 2-phosphoenolpyruvate (PEP) which is essential for photosynthesis. Glyphosate acts as a transition state analog that binds more tightly to the EPSPS-S3P complex than PEP. This binding leads to inhibition of the EPSP synthase's enzymatic catalysis and shuts down the pathway of photosynthesis. Eventually this results in organism death from lack of the essential aromatic amino acids the organism (plant) requires for survival.

A version of the enzyme EPSP synthase that both was resistant to glyphosate and that was still efficient enough to drive adequate plant growth was identified by Monsanto scientists after much trial and error in an *agrobacterium* strain called CP4, which was found surviving in a waste-fed column at a glyphosate production facility. This version of enzyme, CP4 EPSPS, has been engineered into several genetically modified crops to be resistant to glyphosate. This means glyphosate can be used to spray crops to kill weeds and potential disease bacteria without killing the main crop.[ii]

In Humans Glyphosate Primarily Produces:

- **Gut dysbiosis:** It destroys the healthy biome by dysregulating the enzyme pathways. The shikimate-acid pathway in bacteria is essential for us to access certain nutrients.
- **Folate (B9) deficiency**: Folate (B9) is an essential nutrient. Absence of which can lead to numerous pathological effects such as the further production of cysteine to glutathione from homocysteine. Deficiencies lead to hyperhomocysteinemia (excessive protein metabolism, leading to heart disease or circulation problems), gout, vitiligo, macrocytic anemia (blood with insufficient hemoglobin), gingivitis, neural tube defects during pregnancy, cervical dysplasia, inflammatory bowel syndrome (IBS), and others. Reports also indicate that many neuropsychiatric diseases may be secondary to folate (B9) deficiency.
- **DNA/RNA dysregulation:** Disrupts nucleotide formation and DNA and RNA replication which then disrupts normal enzyme production and functionality. This disrupts mitochondrial function and ATP production.
- **Disruption of enzymes:** Essential enzymes needed to digest purines and pyrimidines render the individual nutritionally

deficient: These enzymes are needed to regulate DNA and RNA transcription, protein synthesis, and hormone and neurotransmitter synthesis.

Pesticide and Herbicide: Glyphosate is a pesticide and herbicide used to kill weeds and speed defoliation of "Roundup-Ready" crops for ease of harvest. Spraying GMO crops with glyphosate kills everything growing around it except the GMO plant itself. It is used around the world except in those countries that ban it.[iii] Currently a number of bacteria, insects and weeds are becoming glyphosate resistant by mutating the genetic code for EPSP synthase's need for glycine and substituting the amino acid alanine instead. In order to get the same herbicide and pesticide effect more toxic chemicals are in production. New disease profiles will emerge because of these more toxic chemicals.

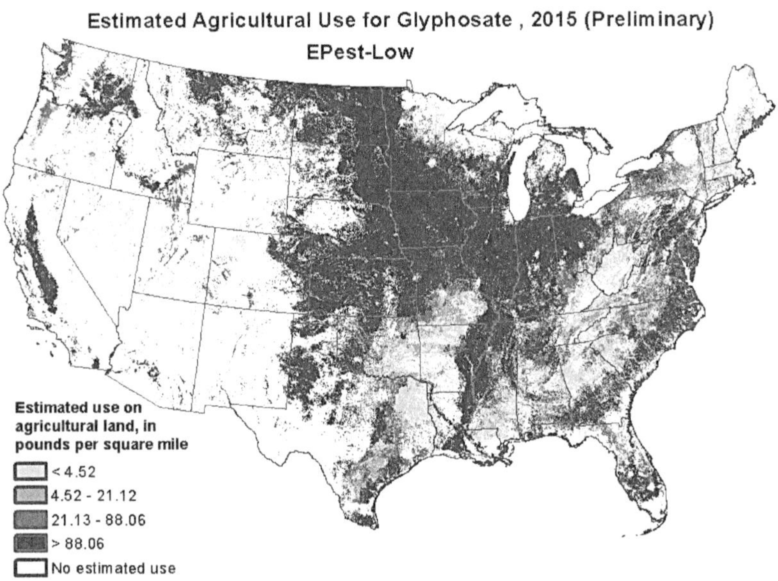

Note: No estimated use means use is not reported. It does not mean there is no use in those areas.

Glyphosate Around the World: Glyphosate was first used in 1974. In 2000 Monsanto's patent on glyphosate expired and use around the world has increased exponentially. In the United States you are at the highest risk of glyphosate toxicity if you live in the agricultural belt of the Midwest due to environmental exposure from aerial drift and ground water contamination.[iv]

If you live in the Midwest or along the Mississippi river, and consume commercially produced wheat, corn and grain-fed animal products, you can be guaranteed to have some degree of glyphosate toxicity. Ground water along the major riverways is contaminated and percolates into all irrigation systems. Health conditions that arise in the planting and harvesting seasons may be a result of exposure. In other parts of the country it may take some time before a diagnosable condition arises.

In May of 2015, the World Health Organization (WHO) classified glyphosate as "probably carcinogenic to humans," based on their review of publicly available research.[v]

Rather than wait for a diagnosis, following a glyphosate free lifestyle will surely ensure your sense of wellbeing.

Top Pesticide Consuming Countries Of The World

Rank	Country	Annual Pesticide Consumption (millions of kilograms)
1	China	1,806
2	United States	386
3	Argentina	265
4	Thailand	87
5	Brazil	76
6	Italy	63
7	France	62
8	Canada	54
9	Japan	52
10	India	40

Usage of Glyphosate by Country: The top countries use of glyphosate is listed in the chart above.[vi] Runners up for high-consuming countries are Turkey, Poland, Taiwan, Columbia, Greece, Portugal, and Lebanon, in that order.[vii] Think about those figs imported from Turkey, Trader Joe's organic imports from China, beef from Brazil (McDonald's) and wheat and lentils from Canada: it is all contaminated with Glyphosate. Every salad dressing with GMO soybean lecithin is contaminated with glyphosate. Soybean lecithin is also used in vaccines as an emulsifier.

Glyphosate in Crops and Livestock: Glyphosate is sprayed on all GMO crops, in people's yards, on school grounds, the sides of the roads, and on all food imported into the United States at the dock yards, including organic foods. Glyphosate is one of the most toxic chemicals to life.[viii] Genetic modification of the crops makes them considered to be 'Roundup-Ready' so they survive when these pesticides are sprayed. Non-GMO crops are sprayed for defoliation for early harvest.

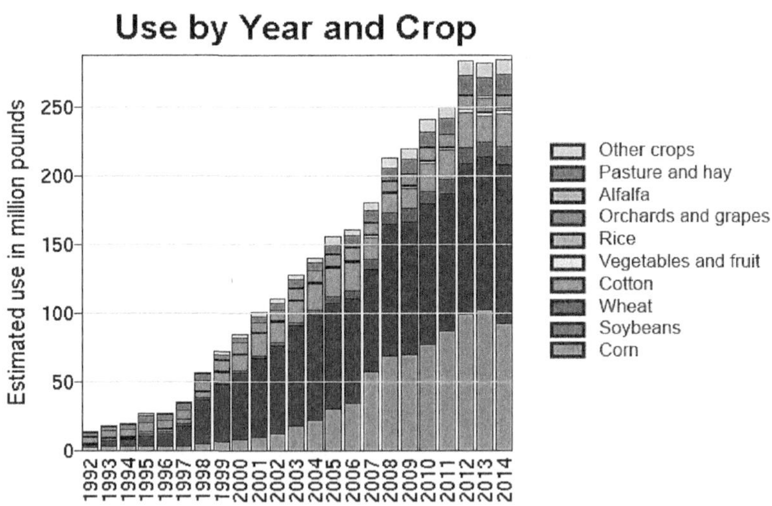

Glyphosate is Found in:

- All GMO crops that are glyphosate resistant and Non-GMO crops where glyphosate is used as a desiccant to force early ripening of the crops and their derivatives: grains, legumes (peas, peanuts, soybeans, lentils), corn, sugar, sugar beets, canola, alfalfa, potatoes, pumpkins, citrus and apples, cotton and sorghum, to name a few.[ix] Also in processed foods like soy lecithin, high-fructose corn syrup, corn starch, etc.
- All non-organically raised meat, dairy, eggs, and poultry as these are fed the above-mentioned foods.
- It is built into the collagen and stored in the fascia, cells, and organs in non-organic grain-fed animals. Fascia is the white fibrous tissue running through all slabs of meat.
- It is also in the GMO soybean-based-feed fed to farm-raised-fish. Accordingly, you will also find it in the fish.

Glyphosate Tolerances in Humans:

- 'Incidental oral exposure' and a chronic Reference Dose (RfD) of 1.75 mg/kg/day based on the NOAEL of 175 mg/ kg/day in the rabbit developmental study.[x]
- Chronic RfD = 1.75 mg/kg/day (US EPA 2006)
- ADI (acceptable daily intake) = 0.3 mg/kg bw (FAO 2000).
- EU limit for drinking water = 0.1 mg/kg (Buffin & Jewell 2001).
- WHO guideline for drinking water = none set.
- Some manufacturers recommend the limit to be between 0.05 and 0.15 mg/kg.
- Independent reviews suggest allowed amount should be no more than 0.025 mg/kg.

Independent reviews of glyphosate found in foods internationally exported from different countries suggest the amount found in those foods is 12 TIMES MORE than the present "acceptable" allowed limit.[xi]

Glyphosate in the Environment: Glyphosate is in our ground water, air, and drinking water, especially in the crop-lands of developed nations around the world where it is used. It is in the food chain from the lowest living entity to the highest and concentrates in each organism as it moves up the food chain. Airborne glyphosate is much easier to poison the body as it readily enters into the body through the membranes of the lungs rather than through the intestinal lining of the digestive system.[xii]

Glyphosate in Vaccines: Vaccines are produced on bovine and porcine nutrient substrates and growth mediums, along with the bovine casein used as nutrition in the incubation process: Gelatin, the basis for all growth mediums, is derived from bone, or other blood derivatives, that are sourced from commercially-fed livestock as such is contaminated.[xiii]

Glyphosate in Organic Food: While we would like to think organic food is free of glyphosate, we are wrong. Testing of organic wines in California, organic foods imported from Turkey,[xiv] Mexico,[xv] China and even those organically-grown in the United States are contaminated by drift from neighboring fields, polluted groundwater, previous soil contamination, contamination during processing in the factory, contamination caused by storage preservatives or from packaging material, and unintentional commingling with conventional goods. It is then also sprayed at the borders prior to entry into the United States.

Glyphosate on Pumpkins: For ease of harvest and as an herbicide glyphosate is sprayed on non-organic pumpkins. While the largest use of these pumpkins is for Halloween, jack-o-lanterns, walking through pumpkin fields to select your pumpkins, or contact with the pumpkins while carving them, will expose your children to high doses of glyphosate.[xvi]

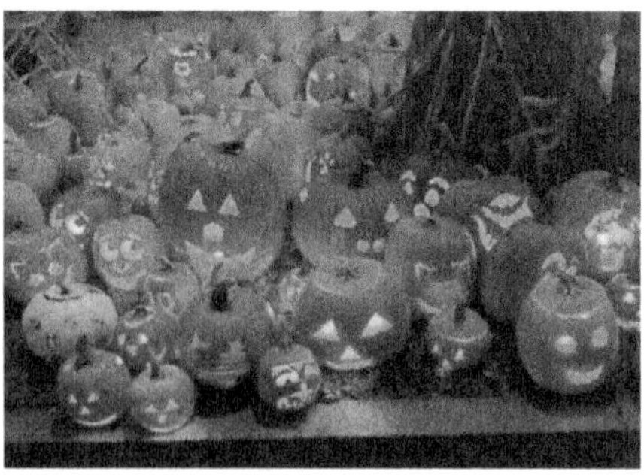

Glyphosate in Cereal: Tests show that glyphosate concentrations in some commercial brand cereals are more that some vitamins and minerals.[xvii] As the food stuff for these cereals are GMO and they are grown on nutritionally dead soil; nutritional content must be synthetically fortified. Both Cheerios and Quaker products are based on oats which are heavily sprayed with glyphosate.

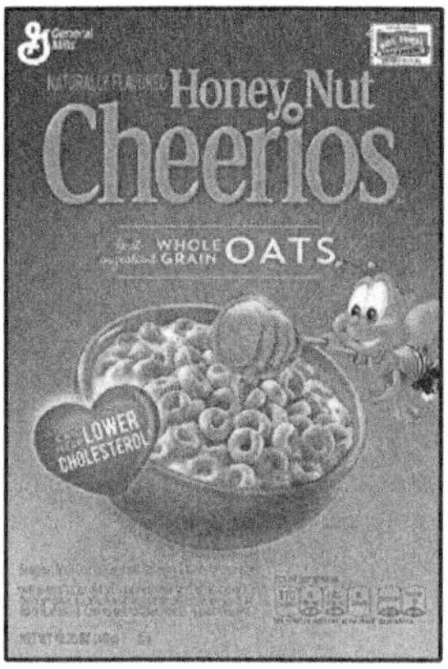

NUTRITION FACTS

Calcium	4600 ppm
Phosphorus	3600 ppm
Magnesium	900 ppm
Vitamin C	320 ppm
Iron	160 ppm
Niacin	140 ppm
Zinc	98 ppm
Vitamin B6	15 ppm
Riboflavin	12 ppm
Thiamin	11 ppm
Folic Acid	7.1 ppm
Vitamin A	3.2 ppm
Glyphosate	0.86 ppm
Vitamin D	0.07 ppm
Vitamin B12	0.02 ppm

NUTRITION FACTS

Phosphorus	4500 ppm
Calcium	2300 ppm
Iron	290 ppm
Vitamin C	160 ppm
Niacin	71 ppm
Zinc	49 ppm
Vitamin E	27 ppm
Folic Acid	7.1 ppm
Vitamin B6	6.1 ppm
Riboflavin	5.8 ppm
Thiamin	5.4 ppm
Glyphosate	2.7 ppm
Vitamin A	1.6 ppm

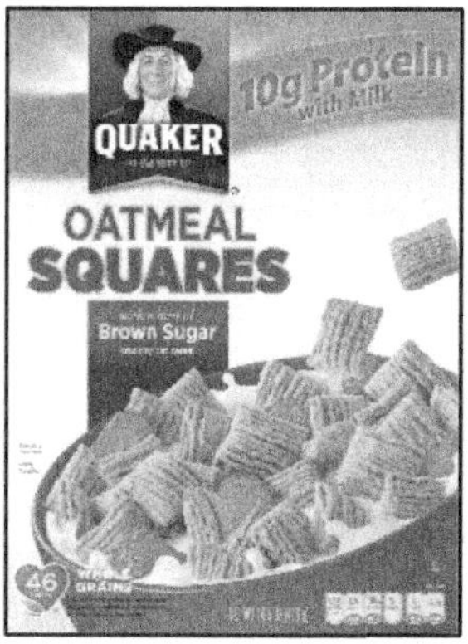

Glyphosate in Wine and Beer: World over, humans like to drink wine and beer. Alcoholic beverages have been a part of human culture for thousands of years and have numerous health benefits if consumed in moderation. Wine and beer are created by the natural fermentation process microorganisms enable. Now, with the general practice of spraying vineyards and hops fields with glyphosate, we are exposed every time we consume an alcoholic beverage. Not only that, as the bacteria, musts, and molds needed for natural fermentation, normally present on grapes or hops, are now destroyed because of glyphosate, they must be artificially added to augment the fermentation process. In California they have found 100% of all wine produced (even organic) to be contaminated.[xviii] This is not only specific to California but all countries that produce wine and use glyphosate. So far, I have found that organic wines in Croatia, Hungary, Italy, and France seem to be fine.

Headaches from drinking wine or beer is a sign that that these are laden with glyphosate. Most hops for beer and the barley for malt is sprayed with glyphosate world over. A study of 14 different brands of German beer found glyphosate levels to exceed allowable limits.[xix] Every time you consume beer, that sleepy feeling is not the alcohol, but rather your liver processing glyphosate. If you are finding you have excess *Candida* conditions from drinking beer, it could be that glyphosate in the beer is destroying your lacto-fermenting-bacteria and driving *Candida* overgrowth.

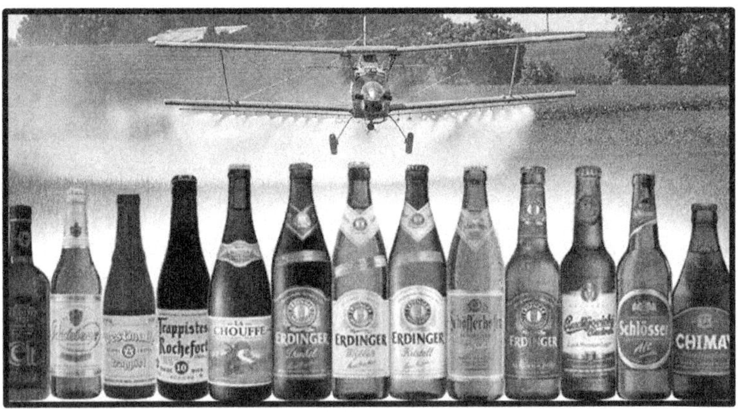

Glyphosate in Honey: The following chart shows the amount of glyphosate found in honey by country. All pollinating crops are dependent upon bees to yield fruit. As bees are non-discriminatory to which flowers they pollinate, they vicariously are collecting glyphosate which gets incorporated into their honey. Moreover, it has been found that contamination for glyphosate affects the homeward navigational system of bees by killing their commensal bacteria. This results in increased collapse of bee colonies (from lost bees) and increased death of the actual bees.[xx] The effect on the bee population world-wide has environmentalists on high alert for the imagined outcome of this trajectory for nature's pollinators.[xxi]

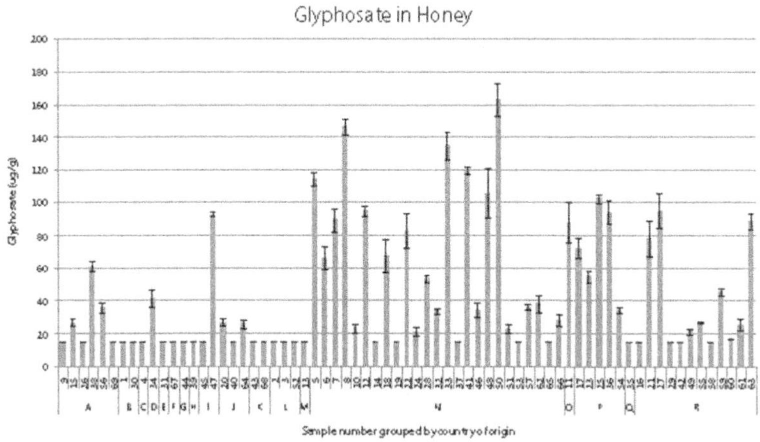

Figure 2: Concentration of glyphosate (ng/g) in honey samples listed by honey origin: (A) Brazil, (B) Canada, (C) China, (D) Germany, (E) Greece, (F) Hungary, (G) India, (H) Korea, (I) blend of Mexico, Brazil, and Uruguay, (J) New Zealand, (K) Spain, (L) Taiwan, (M) blend of Ukraine and Vietnam, (N) USA, (O) blend of SA and Argentina, (P) blend of USA, Argentina and Canada, (Q) blend of USA, South America, (R) unknown origin. Dashed line represents LOQ of method (15 ng/g). Error bars represent concentrations obtained during duplicate analysis.

Glyphosate in Cotton: Most cotton tampons, sanitary pads, and cotton products are contaminated with Glyphosate.[xxii] While we do not ingest cotton: insertion of cotton tampons into the body during menstruation, when mixed with bodily fluids can leach the glyphosate out of the tampon. This glyphosate will kill the naturally occurring lacto-fermenting bacteria in the vagina increasing the risk of yeast infections and through exposure to bodily fluids can become absorbed.

Glyphosate in Tobacco: Tobacco products grown in the United States, Latin America, and South America are heavily sprayed with glyphosate. The children of the farmers of these crops, who live in adjacent housing complexes, show increased risk of congenital microcephaly, epilepsy, delayed motor and mental development, multiple muscular atrophy, and numerous related pathologies.[xxiii]

Glyphosate Poisoning of Pets from Food and Lawn Spraying: Scattered throughout the Midwest of the United States are Purina pet chow silos. Dog and cat foods are found to be chock full of GMO and glyphosate sprayed grain and soy sources. Some samples tested are up to 7.5 % the allowable level for humans.[xxiv] For pets, glyphosate exposure is compounded by direct contact to lawn chemicals and aerial drift from neighboring lawns.[xxv] Such exposure has increased the rates of cancer in dogs (particularly malignant melanomas) in highly contaminated areas, to be equal to that of humans.[xxvi]

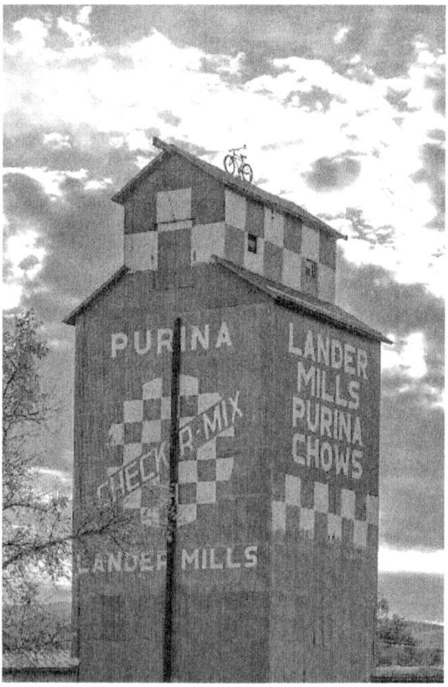

Acute Poisoning from Glyphosate:

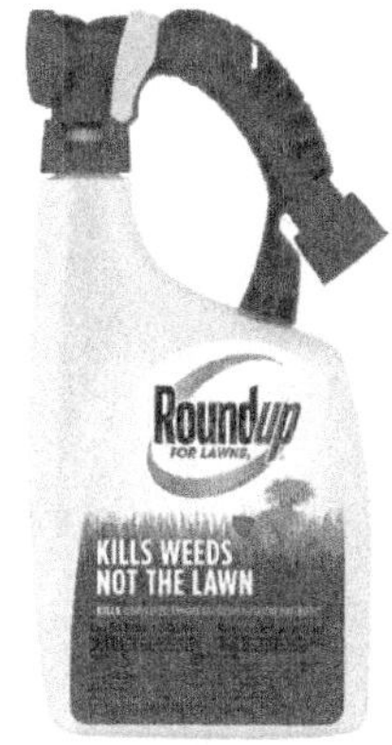

Glyphosate herbicides have been frequently used in self-poisonings and many deaths have occurred, especially in Asia where regulation is minimal. There have also been many cases of unintentional poisonings amongst users and bystanders. Widespread poisonings have occurred in Latin America as a result of aerial spraying of GMO soybean and tobacco crops, and of coca crops in Colombia - effects being recorded as far as 10 km away from the supposed spray zone. The coca spraying (instigated by a US government funded program to eliminate cocaine production in Colombia) has also resulted in widespread animal deaths and food crop losses in the country.[xxvii]

Symptoms of acute poisoning commonly reported from unintentional exposure include vomiting, diarrhea, abdominal pain, gastrointestinal infections, itchy or burning skin, skin rashes and infections (particularly prevalent in children), blisters, burning or weeping eyes, blurred vision, conjunctivitis, headaches, fever, rapid heartbeat, palpitations, raised blood pressure, dizziness, chest pains, numbness, insomnia, depression, debilitation, difficulty in breathing, respiratory infections, dry cough, sore throat, and unpleasant taste or burning in the mouth. Other effects reported include balance disorder (dizziness), reduced cognitive capacity, seizures, impaired vision, smell, hearing and taste, drop in blood pressure, twitches and tics, muscle paralysis, peripheral neuropathy, loss of gross and fine motor skills, excessive perspiration, and severe fatigue.[xxviii]

Comments: Life is Interdependent: no matter where we go, what we do, or what we think, we are all connected. Toxins in one part of the earth affect the rest of the earth.[xxix] We are a part of Creation, made by a plan outside of our comprehension. To think we can tinker with one part of the ecosystem without affecting the whole is narrow-minded, short-sighted, and arrogant. Pollution in my brain affects you and your life because of the actions that pollution causes me to do. We are all cogs in this wheel. In my life, I have chosen the path of non-violence against myself, my fellow human, and this earth that houses me.

I feel my GOD given rights of life, liberty, and happiness have been violated by those who manufacture, use, and create the legislation for the propagation of glyphosate use. I feel like I am living in an inescapable prison when the air I breath, the water I drink, and the food I eat is poisoning me. When my body experiences the symptoms of glyphosate toxicity these feelings of violation grow in me.

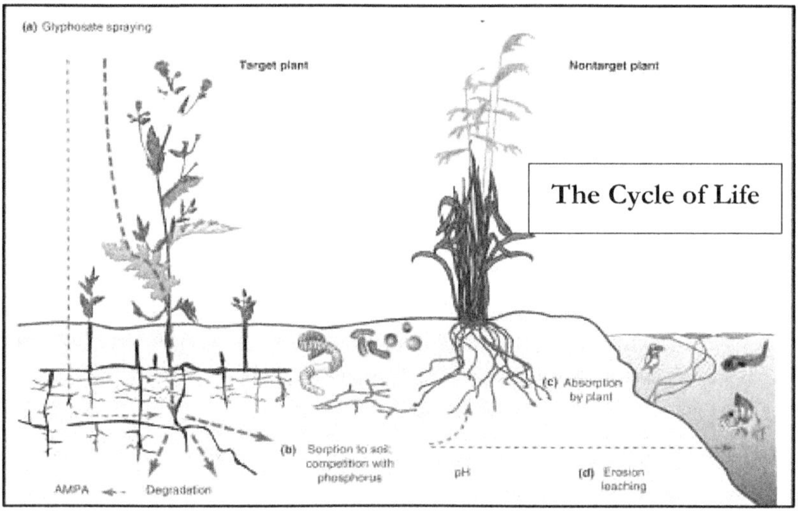

Moreover, when we destroy one part of the environment the trickle up effects compound. For example, possums live in and around farms. They eat ticks, worms, slugs, and snails. They will also eat small rodents and birds. Glyphosate sprayed in the farmlands kills the bacteria housed in these creatures and effects the neurulation process of all creatures with a central nervous system.

Not only does glyphosate effect the reproductive ability of the insects, invertebrates, and amphibians, and the small mammals who also live there, the possums that eat these creatures are now poisoned. But other non- linear effects can happen as well.[xxx] Ticks are a main part of possum diets. Ticks carry a number of diseases, the main one being

Lyme's disease. With reduced possums to eat the ticks, tick populations explode, increasing risk of tick bites in humans. As Glyphosate also suppresses the immune system by occupying adenosine receptor sites, now the newly infected human, with the suppressed immune system, is not able to mount the appropriate immune response to defend itself against the Lyme's invasion and a host of other conditions relating to suppressed immune systems arises. Lyme's disease has increased 101% from 1992 to 2006 (9,908 cases to 19,931), with most cases occurring in children aged 4 to 15 years.[xxxi] Cases increased by 400% from 2000 to 2008.[xxxii]

Can We Stop This? In this instance I do not hold BIG AG alone responsible for this outcome. We are each in our own prison: that of greed from the corporations and the politicians bought and sold for these purposes; that of the farmer's insecurity of providing for his family; and that of the consumer blinded by his nativity, consumption, gluttony, or feelings of unworthiness in his ability to change this trajectory.

None-the-less we need to pay attention, stop purchasing contaminated foods, and stop investing in the companies and the monetary backing that is poisoning the planet. We can grow our own food, support organic farmers, and solicit our legislators. Together we have created this. Together we can change this.

---

i Seneff, S., Morley, W., Hadden, M.J., Michener, M.C. Does glyphosate acting as a glycine analogue contribute to ALS? Journal of. Bioinformatics Proteomics Rev. 2 (2016):1–21.

ii Todd Funke, Huijong Han, Martha L. Healy-Fried, Markus Fischer, and Ernst Schönbrunn. Molecular basis for the herbicide resistance of Roundup-Ready crops. Proceedings of the National Academy of Sciences of the United States of America. 2006 Aug 29; 103(35): 13010–13015. https://www.ncbi.nlm.nih.gov/pmc/articles/PMC1559744/.

iii Glyphosate Bans and Restrictions Across the Globe. March 25, 2015. http://responsibletechnology.org/irtnew/wp-content/uploads/2016/01/2-Glyphosate-Bans-and-Restrictions-Across-the-Globe.pdf.

iv Pariona, Amber. USCA Pesticide National Synthesis Project. https://water.usgs.gov/nawqa/pnsp/usage/maps/show_map.php?year=2015&map=GLYPHOSATE&hilo=L.

v Corbin Hiar. Under fire by U.S. politicians, World Health Organization defends its claim that an herbicide causes cancer. E&E News. Feb. 7, 2018. https://www.sciencemag.org/news/2018/02/who-rebuts-house-committee-criticisms-about-glyphosate-cancer-warning.

vi World Atlas. 2017. https://www.worldatlas.com/articles/top-pesticide-consuming-countries-of-the-world.html.

vii Mitra, Tony. Exploring citizens duty on food security, & environmental sustainability issues. 2017. http://www.tonu.org/2017/01/24/charts/.

viii Seneff, Stephanie. Multiple articles and research on glyphosate, autism, obesity, celiac disease and more. http://people.csail.mit.edu/seneff/.

ix USCA Pesticide National Synthesis project. https://water.usgs.gov/nawqa/pnsp/usage/maps/show_map.php?year=2015&map=GLYPHOSATE&hilo=L.

x Glyphosate. National Toxic Encephalopathy Foundation. http://www.national-toxic-encephalopathy-foundation.org/roundup.pdf.

xi Jill. Europe's Top 5 Glyphosate Herbicide Toxic Countries. https://www.moyoway.com/europes-top-5-glyphosate-herbicide-toxic-countries.html.

xii Ji, Sayer. Roundup Weed killer found in 75% of rain samples, Gov. Study Finds. GreenMed Pub. Feb. 2014. http://www.greenmedinfo.com/blog/roundup-weedkiller-found-75-air-and-rain-samples-gov-study-finds/.

xiii Honeycutt, Zen. Glyphosate in Vaccines Report. Moms Across America. Sept 2016. https://d3n8a8pro7vhmx.cloudfront.net/yesmaam/pages/1707/attachments/original/1473130173/FullGlyphosateinVaccinesReport_(6).pdf?1473130173.

xivxiv Bernhard Speiser, Sena Ertem, Elisabeth Rüegg, Beate Huber Beate. Survey of the Residue Situation in Turkish Organic Products. ARGE FiBL Türkei. German-Turkish Cooperation Organic Agriculture. (2013). http://orgprints.org/25032/1/speiser-etal-2014-turkey-residueSurvey-report.pdf.

xv Mexico: The dangers of industrial corn and its processed edible products. GRAIN | 20 March 2018 | Against the grain, Seeds. https://www.grain.org/article/entries/5906-mexico-the-dangers-of-industrial-corn-and-its-processed-edible-products.

xvi Nathan Johanning. Weed Management in Cucurbits. University of Illinois Extension Murphysboro. Illinois. https://jhawkins54.typepad.com/files/weed-management-in-cucurbits---johanning.pdf.

xvii Alex Formuzis.Tests Reveal more Weed Killer then Some Vitamins in Kids Cereals. Environmental Working Group. October 31, 2018. https://www.ewg.org/release/tests-reveal-more-weed-killer-some-vitamins-kids-cereals?

xviii Roundup's Toxic Chemical Glyphosate Found in 100% of California Wines Tested. Feb 28, 2018. WineWaterWatch.org. http://winewaterwatch.org/2018/02/roundups-toxic-chemical-glyphosate-found-in-100-of-california-wines-tested/.

xix German Beer Industry in Shock Over Monsanto Glyphosate Contamination. Sustainable Pulse 25 February 2016. https://www.globalresearch.ca/german-beer-industry-in-shock-over-glyphosate-contamination/5633850.

xx María Sol Balbuena, Léa Tison, Marie-Luise Hahn, Uwe Greggers, Randolf Menzel, Walter M. Farina. Effects of sublethal doses of glyphosate on honeybee navigation. Journal of Experimental Biology 2015 218: 2799-2805; doi: 10.1242/jeb.117291.

xxi Rubio, Abraxis, Guo, Emily. Kamp, Lisa. Survey of Glyphosate Residues in Honey, Corn and Soy Products. Journal of Environmental & Analytical Toxicity. October 2, 2014. https://www.omicsonline.org/open-access/survey-of-glyphosate-residues-in-honey-corn-and-soy-products-2161-0525.1000249.php?aid=36354.

xxii Tampons, sterile cotton, sanitary pads contaminated with glyphosate – study. 23 Oct. 2015. https://www.rt.com/usa/319524-tampons-cotton-glyphosate-monsanto/.

xxiii GMO Kids? Argentina Moms Confront Monsanto and Philip Morris Over Greed and Pesticides. Organic Consumers Association. July 17, 2018. https://www.organicconsumers.org/blog/monsanto-roundup-gmos-argentina.

xxiv Jiang Zhao, Steven Pacenk, Jing Wuc, Brian K. Richards, Tammo Steenhuis, Kenneth Simpson, Anthony G. Haya. Detection of glyphosate residues in companion animal feeds. Environmental Pollution Volume 243, Part B, December 2018.

https://www.sciencedirect.com/science/article/pii/S0269749118319067.

xxv Is Your Pet Exposed to Glyphosate? New Study to Offer Tests and Investigate Risks. Organic Consumers Association. May. 29, 2018. https://www.ecowatch.com/glyphosate-pet-health-2573246280.html.

xxvi Ibid.

xxvii Glyphosate. National toxic encephalopathy foundation. http://www.national-toxic-encephalopathy-foundation.org/roundup.pdf.

xxviii Ibid.

xxix Augustenborg, Dr. Cara. Earth Care, People Care, Future Care: Permaculture. Glyphosate License - Sneaked past by EU during the UK Brexit week. July 2016.

https://www.permaculture.co.uk/news/14678071247345/glyphosate-license-sneaked-past-eu-during-uk-brexit-week.

xxx Agustín Estrada-Peña, José de la Fuente, Richard S. Ostfeld, Alejandro Cabezas-Cruz. Interactions between tick and transmitted pathogens evolved to minimise competition through nested and coherent networks. Scientific Reports volume5, Article number: 10361 (2015).

xxxi Incidence rates of certain tick-borne diseases on the rise in US Experts discuss reasons for the increase and review prevention techniques. Infectious Diseases in Children, April 2012. https://www.healio.com/pediatrics/news/print/infectious-diseases-in-children/%7B91e4d235-1090-417d-8b2d-ec47a1f0cb94%7D/incidence-rates-of-certain-tick-borne-diseases-on-the-rise-in-us.

xxxii Ibid.

2. The Primordial Sea

Protons, neutrons, and electrons make up the elements of the natural world. The periodic table maps out these elements according to their differences and similarities. Through the laws of chemistry, certain elements naturally bind with other elements. Abiogenesis, informally the 'Origin of Life,' is the natural process whereby life arose from non-living matter, such as simple organic compounds.

Carbon is the fundamental element all life systems on this earth are based upon. Carbon, catalyzed by the electron charges of metals, in relationship to the elements, hydrogen, oxygen and nitrogen, forms simple amino acids. Nitrogen self-organizes with hydrogen and oxygen to form the five and six ringed nucleotides which make up the nitrogenous bases of deoxyribonucleic acid (DNA) and ribonucleic acid (RNA). These strands pair and swirl in the primordial sea of elements coding for all possible proteins in all life forms.

Joseph Moran, a young scientist, set himself upon the task to see if he could recreate the presumed conditions leading up to life on this planet. His lab found that mixing metals in water, under a pressurized atmosphere of carbon dioxide produced acetate (acetic acid with an earth or metal element attached) and pyruvate, an intermediate and an end-product, respectively, of the acetyl coenzyme A metabolic pathway (Krebs cycle). Exposing pyruvate to the same conditions plus hydrazine

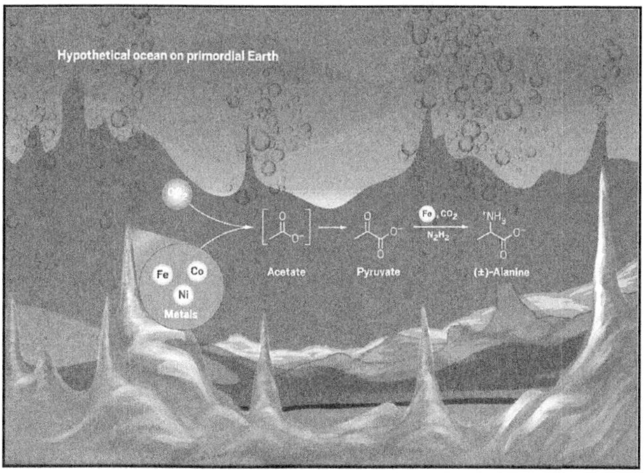

gives the amino acid alanine. The researchers believe these reactions illustrated the plausible prebiotic pathways used to create the complex molecules necessary for life to establish itself.[xxxiii, xxxiv]

Protein chains of amino acids assemble according to the same laws of attraction between elements. The functionality and replication of these proteins and nucleic acid strands are by nature, self-regulated through built in feedback loops.

According to the abiogenesis theory, proteins formed to create structure, and the simplest enzymes, neurotransmitters, and hormones that worked together in self-regulating circular feedback loops optimize the DNA directives that coded them. Phospholipid cell membranes formed around clusters of DNA strands and the first living organism came into existence.

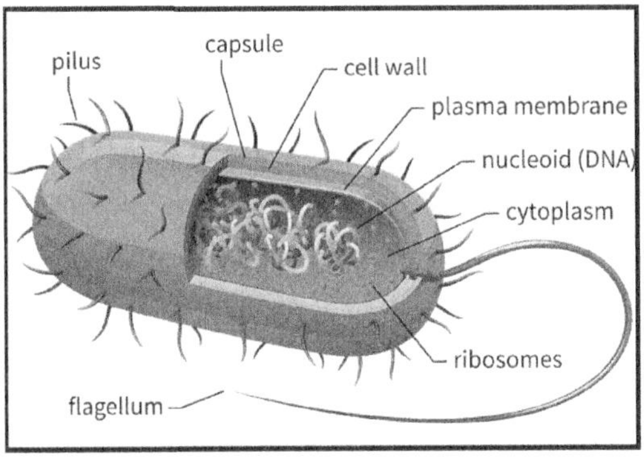

The simplest living organisms are single celled prokaryotes. Prokaryotes include bacteria and cyanobacteria. These single cell organisms process a variety of functions based on the environment they inhabit, and the subsequent editing of the genetic code in their DNA. These organisms were the first to produce oxygen during photosynthesis, which has allowed all other living organisms to come into existence.

As the DNA code became more and more complex the resultant living organisms, too became more complex. Eukaryotes formed by engulfing single celled bacteria, which then serve as the mitochondria of these more advanced cells. Through the cellular respiration (Krebs cycle) that takes place in the mitochondria, ATP is produced. ATP is the functional unit for energy which drives enzymatic functionality, and all metabolic and detoxification processes.

Over time as more complex living organisms evolved, species developed and at some point, approximately 200,000 years ago, Man emerged. Man, as a conscious being. Man as a complex DNA replication system, not separate from the earth, nature's laws or the single celled bacteria that are housed in his body. Man, whose consciousness, thought forms, metabolic processes, immune system regulation, hormonal and neurotransmitter production are a direct function of his relationship to the commensal bacteria that populate his intestinal lining. And that when aligned in himself in relationship to nature and these bacteria, his vital force and expression of the immune system is the direct manifestation of the vital force of the bacteria he houses. Man, capable of rendering the finest music, scholarly achievements, and global exploration, is the same Man stricken by poverty, perversion, and war. Bacterial populations vary in different cultures based upon the food he eats, the wine he drinks, and the medicine he chooses.

According to The Book of Genesis, GOD created the Heavens and the Earth. On the earth He separated the water and dry land. He populated the land and the waters with all the living creatures of this existence. Then He created Man in his own image: a reflection of the self-organizing, self-generating, self-regulating, and self-correcting quality of nature.

Comments: It is not my intention in this essay to stir religious, theosophical, or scientific debate with these two versions of Creation but rather to point out their common theme. That is, within everything is GOD. GOD is the **Generating-Organizing-Delivering/Destroying system** that governs how chemicals interact with each other and how Man rectifies his conscience: the built-in self-regulating aspect of thought and action. The energy of Creation is the unified field and living entities in this field replicate under the laws reflected in the Golden Ratio.

> "The solution to infinite non-destructive (charge) compression IS the unified field. Perfect compression within that field is the solution to virtually every science problem in history: gravity, alchemy, fusion, urban design,

computers, the physics of human (peak) perception/bliss; the list goes on. What this means then is that we have just proven the theory of wave mechanics showing that the golden ratio IS the solution to perfect (charge) compression" (Albert Einstein).[xxxv]

The charged field of nature governs not only the earth upon which we live and the food which we eat but also our physical body and our conscious existence. The critical regulation of DNA replication and transcription is held in exquisite balance by this very force. Everything in this system is precisely ordered by the holy and sacred force that is life. GOD is truth. GOD is love. GOD is consciousness. GOD is the blueprint of life by which the vital force connects to and maintains all living beings. With consciousness comes conscience and the ability to realize truth. This truth can be seen in the self-organizing patterns we see in nature and in our body and mind. When we realize who we really are we have GOD-consciousness and connection to the entire universe.

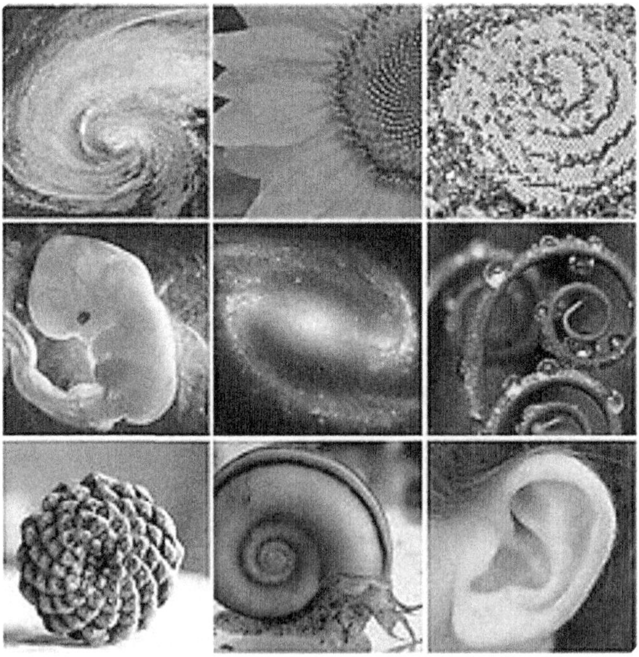

In this existence we have been given free will to live in accordance to the grand blueprint or not. If we step outside of our personal agendas, into pure consciousness, as directed by pure conscience, we find oneness and connection to truth and can live in the moment in pure bliss. Here only we can truly experience the unified field. Through the laws of nature, we have evolved, and if we live in accordance to those laws of nature, we will be healthy in our body as all systems can learn and adapt because of the innate self-correcting feedback loops that want to keep us operating in complete order. As like conscience, once we are aware of our errs, we correct our actions. Thus, to live in truth we are beholden to willingly live in accordance to nature's plan. Because the blueprint of Creation is encrypted in us as well, we have a reference point from which to operate.

Mystics have contemplated the origin of human consciousness since they became aware of their own consciousness. Yet, many have found no conclusive understanding as to what consciousness is. With respect to glyphosate, among other things, it seems the human animal is not yet so evolved, as to fully comprehend the complexity of his biological existence nor the ramifications of his will or actions. Or, he has devolved and forgotten, or chooses not to oblige his conscience, either individually or collectively.

Glyphosate's main target is the single celled bacteria (also mitochondrial function): the foundational living unit of all living systems. The idea that we can use glyphosate to kill our perceived pests (bacteria and single-celled organisms) without fully comprehending the ramifications on the ecosystem and our biological system is mis-guided thinking. We are not separate from nature, and we are not here to manipulate it to our contrivances. To think that we can take it upon ourselves to tinker with the code of life through genetic manipulation of the food we eat without first understanding what life is, what consciousness is and how it works, is a violation of our built-in conscience mechanism.

The individual consumer of foods contaminated with glyphosate may not have begun to consider what might be in his food, let alone reflect upon the significance of the connection between his consciousness, conscience, GOD, and the natural laws of chemistry governing the physiological functions of his body. None-the-less, if he neglects to be conscious about what he puts in his mouth and has misconceptions about this existence, eventually his body will succumb to a number of health issues without him understanding why.

The conventional doctor, who is also uninformed, would willingly prescribe antibiotics, antivirals, fertility drugs, serotonin reuptake inhibitors, antihistamines, or chemotherapy in attempts to address the issues that have arisen. Neither of them will understand why the therapies fail to work, unless they had a predilection towards the basic understanding that we are what we eat, and our food is contaminated.

In writing this essay, as I am searching how to solve this problem, I ask, what is needed to further awaken human consciousness with respect to the laws that govern the body? I ask what is needed in my own consciousness to come to terms with the reality of toxins all around me? I ask how can we call upon nature's processes for healing to pull humanity back from the brink of self-annihilation? This is not only for the care of our physical body, but also with regards to bringing consciousness to the human thought forms that drive the destruction of the environment and the individuals who choose to partake in the global economic structures that maintain this trajectory.

---

xxxiii Tien Nguyen. Joseph Moran. Origins explorer is seeking the chemistry that sparked life on Earth. Chemical Engineering News, August 20, 2018. Volume 96, Issue 33.

xxxiv Photo Credit: Yang H. Ku/C&EN/Shutterstock.

xxxv Einstein, Albert. Implosion Group's website about Dan Winter- Sacred Geometry & Coherent Emotion, & Heart Tuner + Bliss Tuner. http://goldenmean.info/.

3. Glyphosate and DNA and RNA Basics

Nucleotides are biopolymers essential to all life: they are formed with a 5-carbon-ring sugar, a phosphate group and a nitrogenous base: purine (double-5-nitrogen ring) or pyrimidine (6-nitrogen-ring)). If the sugar molecule is ribose the polymer is RNA: if it is deoxyribose, then the polymer is DNA.

Nucleic acids (chains of nucleotides) are found in all living things. They encode function and store information in the nucleus of every life form on earth from the smallest bacteria to the most sophisticated mammal. That which is encoded in the DNA is the blueprint of life.

The nitrogenous bases are guanine, cytosine, adenine, thymine, and uracil. These bind with a single sugar ribose and phosphate group to form the nucleotides guanosine, cytidine, adenosine, and uridine in RNA (G-C-A-U). In DNA they bind with a deoxyribose and phosphate to form deoxyguanosine, deoxycytidine, deoxyadenosine, and thymidine respectively (G-C-A-T).

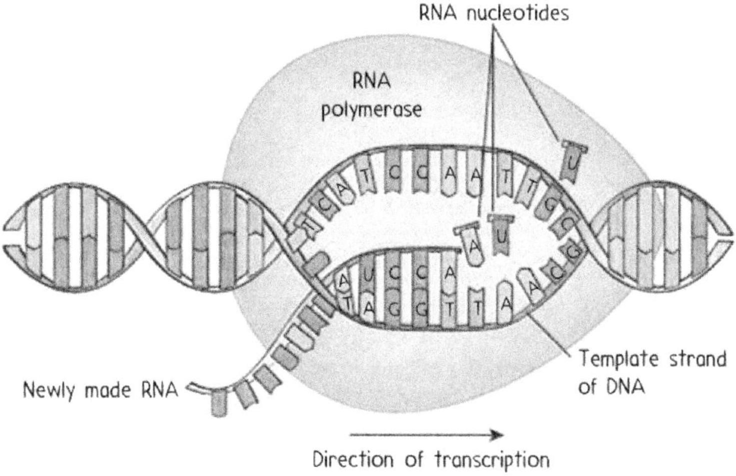

Glyphosate inteferes with creation of nucleotides:[xxxvi] DNA codes for RNA transcription and RNA reads the DNA and codes for protein synthesis through base pair combinations. A pairs with T in DNA and U in RNA. C pairs with G in both. Nucleotides are strung together from free purine and pyrimidine nitrogenous units in the intercellular fluids the transcription takes place in. The amino acid glycine is the scaffold upon which the purine bases or adenine and guanine are formed. Glyphosate has a stronger polarization and chemostatic potential than glycine (migratory potential across membranes, in response to electromagnetic differentials). If cellular fluids are contaminated with glyphosate, access to glycine becomes limited, thus interrupting the formation of purine based nucleotides.

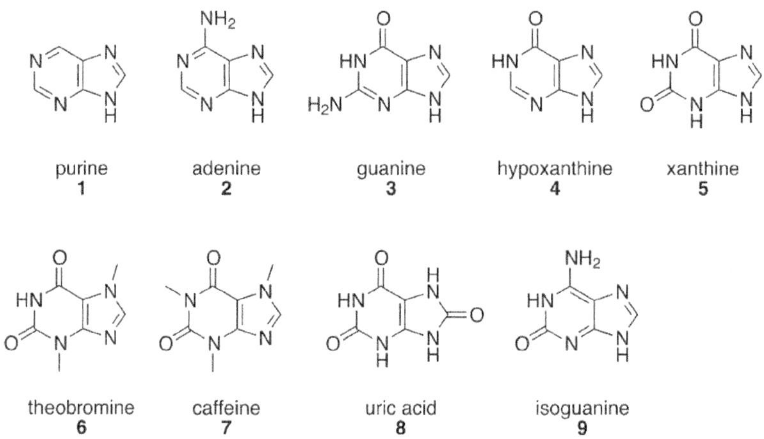

Some Purines

Glyphosate Affects Purinergic Signaling of the Immune System and Neurotransmitters:[xxxvii] The purine bases of RNA are guanine and adenine which form guanosine and adenosine respectively, which are both glycine dependent. Each interact with their specific receptor sites in cell membranes. The pyrimidine bases formed are cytosine, thiamine, and uracil. Purines and pyrimidines are signaling agents that act as antagonists to each other in various functions by engaging with these receptor sites throughout living organisms. In humans, purinergic signaling to the immune system inhibits and activates many different cell types, regulates neurotransmitter and hormonal function, and specific cellular receptor sites in various organs and glands throughout the body.

This signaling process is based on chemical gradient scales of different interrelated factors and is reflective of the blueprints' prerogative. Relative concentrations of purines and pyrimidines are self-inhibiting and self-activating based on their own feedback loops. They work in balance with each other to inhibit or activate DNA replication and RNA transcription. Purines and pyrimidines are also responsible for functionality of enzymes. As glyphosate interferes with nucleotide synthesis, specifically the purines that need glycine, the critical balance between purines and pyrimidines is altered. An imbalance in their ratios will have a direct effect on functionality and expression of the enzymes and regulatory processes they govern.

Purinergic Signaling Molecules Play a Role in:

- Critical regulation of the immune system through interaction with G-protein coupled receptor sites (guanine-nucleotide binding proteins (GPCR)) in cell membranes: white blood cell activity, activation or suppression, and healthy immune system response towards infectious disease or cancer cell lines respectively.
- Cellular respiration (Krebs cycle) to produce ATP (adenosine triphosphate).
- Endocrine function with regards to intraglandular communication and the stimulation or suppression of hormone synthesis.
- Neurotransmitter production and function: tryptophan - precursory function to: serotonin (wellbeing and happiness), melatonin (sleep inducer), glutamate (excitatory), GABA (inhibitory in the mature brain- memory and learning, excitatory in the developing brain) and dopamine (pleasure response).
- Heart and respiratory function (dilation and constriction).
- Detoxification pathways (methylation and glutathione production).

Glyphosates' Relationship to Adenosine: With the purine base of adenine, adenosine is of import with respect to adenosine triphosphate (ATP) production and subsequent reduction and the purinergic signaling to the receptor sites listed below. Glyphosate interferes with the production of ATP and the enzyme (adenosine deaminase (ADA)) both needed to reduce adenosine to inosine, which plays a role in DNA and RNA editing. Altered adenosine concentrations produce inflammatory responses and neurotransmitter dysregulation. Reduction in ATP production through interrupted glycolysis (cellular respiration). Glyphosates main target is cessation of cellular respiration which leads to an excess of adenosine, producing excessive sleepiness and suppression of the immune system through activation of the adenosine receptor sites.

Glyphosate Driven Vitamin and Mineral Deficiencies Affect ATP and Adenosine Levels: [xxxviii] While insufficient production of intracellular adenosine (through faulty glycine dependent scaffolds) and the secondary results of improper DNA transcription and protein synthesis leads to one set of problems, insufficient breakdown of excess adenosine leads to another set of issues.

Adenosine Triphosphate (ATP): In all living organisms ATP is produced in the mitochondria for all intra- and extra- cellular functions. Adenosine is responsible for all cellular energy in the form of adenosine triphosphate (ATP). ATP is formed through cellular respiration in the Krebs cycle in animals and photosynthesis in plants.[xxxix] Glyphosate is used as a defoliant because it interferes with photosynthesis which is how plants generate ATP. As a pesticide it interferes with the mitochondria's ability to produce ATP. Glyphosate's purpose is to render cell death. As glyphosate interferes with the functioning of all mitochondria, it follows that human cell death will also occur at higher concentrations. Reduction in ATP production reduces the energy available for all enzymatic and cellular processes.

During glyphosate metabolism, several intermediaries are formed: aminomethylphosphonic acid (AMPA), methylphosphonic acid, and N-(phosphonomethyl)iminodiacetic acid (PMIDA). It is these byproducts produced in the metabolism of glyphosate that reduces cellular levels of

ATP and increases cell death.[xl] Decreased cellular respiration means that the energy needed for all other cellular functions is also reduced.

Adenosine Deaminase (ADA): Once ATP is formed through glycolysis it is utilized for energy. It is the liberation of the phosphate groups that releases energy to be used for other cellular processes: DNA transcription, protein synthesis, and enzymatic functionality. In this process ATP is reduced to ADP (adenosine diphosphate) and then further reduced to adenosine once again. ADA is needed to further reduce adenosine to inosine (an antioxidant and peroxynitrate scavenger). ADA is dependent on molybdenum and cobalamin (B12) which can become deficient in glyphosate toxicity. Deficiency of ADA, from a glyphosate induced cobalamin (B12) and/or molybdenum deficiency, can lead to an excess of free adenosine in extracellular tissue which forces occupation of the adenosine receptor sites resulting in elevated IgE antibodies (elevated allergic response), immunological suppression, activation of RNA viruses, cytokine storms, cancer cell proliferation and tumor metastasis.[xli, xlii]

Glyphosate Driven ADA Deficiency and Allergic Responses: An ADA deficiency leads to activation of adenosine receptor sites which serves to elevate IgE antibodies to a number of potential food based allergens.[xliii] IgE has an essential role in Type I Hypersensitivity, which results in the activation of mast cells, located in the fascia (collagen), which, once activated by IgE, degranulate and release histamine. ADA deficiency coupled with adenosine receptor sites being activated (see below) can result in various allergic diseases such as allergic asthma, most types of sinusitis, allergic rhinitis, food allergies, mast cell activation disease, and specific types of chronic urticaria and atopic dermatitis.[xliv] Exposure to glyphosate-rich air samples as well as glyphosate alone to the lungs increased: eosinophil and neutrophil counts, and mast cell degranulation by activating the A3 receptor sites.[xlv]

Excess Adenosine Activates Adenosine Receptor Sites: A result of ADA deficiency is excess of adenosine. In human cells, extracellular adenosine binds with adenosine receptor sites on surface membranes that stimulate specific activities. These adenosine receptor sites are in the neural membrane, heart cells, and in the peripheral mucous membranes of the lungs and digestive track. Correspondingly these sites regulate heart, lungs, immune system, and neurotransmitter function.

Adenosine acts as an agonist on these receptor sites: A1, A2a, A2b, A3. Because glyphosate induces higher adenosine levels, the afore mentioned conditions are the result. The following receptor sites will be upregulated or down regulated depending.

- **A1**: Bronchospasm and decreased heart rate, arteriolar constriction in the kidney. Sleep inducing.
- **A2a**: Vasodilation of the heart, increases oxygen levels, decreases in dopamine levels: this receptor site works in opposition to A2b. Insomnia inducing.
- **A2b**: Release of calcium, bronchospasm.
- **A3**: Contraction of the smooth muscles of blood vessels and heart muscle relaxation. Inhibition of neutrophil degranulation. Stimulation of mast cell degranulation and eosinophil proliferation.

Each receptor site type is responsible for a specific function. Other purine bases, theobromine (chocolate,) and caffeine, for example, are adenosine antagonists (have the opposite effect) on these same receptor sites. This means they counteract the action of adenosine.

Adenosine is directly related to dopamine levels and sleep through its engagement with A2a receptor sites. Excess in adenosine leads to a reduction in dopamine and increase in wakefulness. Dopamine is also the neurotransmitter of the pleasure response.

Glyphosate's Disruption of the Biome Changes Adenosine Levels in Perinatal Development:[xlvi] In pregnancy and the first two years of life adenosine levels are intended to be high so as to naturally suppress the immune system so the baby is not miscarried and the infant's immune system can establish itself without becoming over-reactive to the normal lacto-fermenting bacteria in the mother's biome. Disruption of the gut biome of the mother and infant by glyphosate leads to elevated adenosine levels and resultant changes in immune system function and neurotransmitter regulation in the infant. An over-reactive immune system response leads to excessive histamine production and allergic response in relation to the normal lacto-fermenting bacteria. Glyphosate disruption of the enzymes that help to breakdown lactic acid results in lactic acidosis, a condition marked by elevated histamine levels. Elevated lactic acid and heightened histamine can lead to cerebral inflammation, developmental delays, autism, and changes in mood and behavior.

Glyphosate Driven Elevated Extracellular Adenosine Levels: In non-reproducing adults, elevated adenosine leads to immune system suppression and increases the tendency towards cancer cell and tumor growths. Glyphosate driven elevated adenosine levels suppresses healthy T cell proliferation and cytokine activity:[xlvii] Killer T cells are needed to destroy cancer cells.

Glyphosate Interferes with DNA and RNA Editing:[xlviii] The zinc dependent enzyme adenosine deaminase (ADA) is responsible for the reduction of adenosine to inosine which plays in the vital role of RNA editing. Glyphosate causes a reduction in and alters the form of ADA. There is a feedback loop in healthy ADA driven RNA editing that regulates the form of ADA expression. This feedback loop governs all gene coding and either activates the development of gene mutations and cancer cells or checks them. Elevated levels of copper, silver, or mercury inhibit ADA. Proliferation of RNA retroviruses results.

Glyphosate and Guanine-Protein Coupled Receptor Sites (GPCRs): This is large guanine dependent protein family of receptors that direct molecules between cells and activate internal signal transduction pathways and cellular responses (purinergic signaling system). Many of these receptor sites are metal and calcium dependent (Ligand binding sites and Calcium channels respectively).

There are two principal signal transduction pathways involving GPCR sites:

- **The cAMP signal pathway:** the cAMP pathway is a derivative of adenosine triphosphate (ATP) and is used for intracellular signal transduction for activating enzymes, lipids, other GPCR sites, transcription factors for DNA and RNA gene functions, regulating catecholamines (neurotransmitters derived from tyrosine), and hormones.

- **The phosphatidylinositol signal pathway:** phosphoinositides play important roles in lipid signaling, cell signaling, and membrane trafficking. These receptor sites are present in all cell membranes.

Healthy operation of GPCR sites are vital for the functionality of all target organ systems and functions. More importantly, the functionality of these receptor sites are deleteriously impacted by glyphosate toxicity.[xlix, l]

These intermembrane receptor sites are categorized into the following groups and functions:

Class A, Rhodopsin-like: these cover a wide range of functions including various autonomic neurotransmitter and hormonal processes susceptible to and regulated by a photoisomerization reaction (a reaction triggered by light) to translate electromagnetic radiation from the environment into cellular signals. The action of these sites is triggered by the environment we live in. They are influenced by touch, taste, smell, temperature, visual stimulus, the sun, moon, and stars. These sites are on all surface membranes and coverings of the body as well as on many organ cells. These sites connect us to, and are activated by, the world we live in and allow us to experience beauty in life. For example, sites on the pineal gland are activated or suppressed by sunlight, cosmic and telluric influences, and mental or emotional stimuli. For example, being hugged by a loved one releases oxytocin and a cascade of other

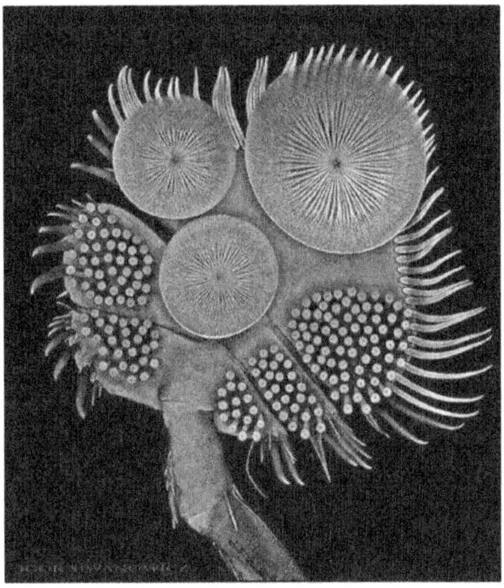

Rhodopsin receptor sites on a beetles' foot

hormones and neurotransmitters creating the experience of love and wellbeing.

Class B, Secretin receptor family: many secretin receptors are regulated by peptide hormones from the glucagon hormone family affecting endocrine system and function. For example, vasoactive intestinal peptide receptors and receptors for secretin, calcitonin, vasopressin, and parathyroid hormone/parathyroid hormone-related peptides. These receptors sites are activated by hormones implicit to the hypothalamic-pituitary-adrenal and hypothalamic-pituitary-thyroid axes.

Class C, Metabotropic glutamate/pheromone: receptors that bind with glutamate, an amino acid that functions as an excitatory neurotransmitter.

Class D, Fungal mating pheromone receptors: not relevant in humans but are receptors on the membranes of *Saccharomyces cervisiae.*

Class E, Cyclic AMP receptors: cAMP and its associated kinases (enzymes) function in several biochemical processes, including the regulation of glycogen, sugar, and lipid metabolism, and transferring into cells the effects of hormones like glucagon and adrenaline, which cannot pass through the plasma membrane; also, activation of calcium channels. Thus, cAMP pathways are utilized in bacteria for transcriptions of enzymes. The cAMP pathways regulate genes that govern cancer expression and disorders of the cerebral cortex. Sperm motility is directly related to calcitonin's action on its cAMP pathways.

Class F, Frizzled/Smoothened: Frizzled protein or smooth receptors also play key roles in governing cell polarity, embryonic development, formation of the neural tube, neural synapses, cell proliferation, and many other processes in developing and adult organisms.

Implications of Glyphosate on GPCR Functionality:

i. G-protein coupled receptors in the mammalian brain bind several different neurotransmitters, including serotonin, dopamine, GABA, and glutamate, all affecting behavioral and mood regulation. Glyphosate driven alterations in functionality of these receptors change mood, social, and cognitive expression.[li]

ii. Glyphosate causes malfunctioning in the glycine and calcium dependent glutamate GPCR sites.[lii]

iii. Chemokine receptors bind ligands (metal plus an ion = electron donner) that mediate intercellular communication between cells of the immune system. GPCR sites, such as histamine receptors, bind inflammatory agents which activates signaling of target cells in the inflammatory response. Glyphosate acts as a chelator and binds with the trace metals cobalt, iron, copper, molybdenum, manganese, and zinc which are needed for these receptors to function properly: [liii] thus, interfering with their important role in the GPCR site's functionality. The ions that bind and activate metal dependent neurotransmitter GPCR sites include light-sensitive compounds, odors, hormones, pheromones, and neurotransmitters.[liv]

iv. GPCRs are also involved in immune-modulation and are directly involved in upregulation of Toll-Like-Receptor (TLR)-induced immune responses from T cells and mast cells to microbial agents. These sites govern regulation of immune system activity and inflammation.[lv] Glyphosate driven upregulation of these sites increases cytokine activity and a resultant systemic inflammation. While normal human exposure to commensal microbial agents down regulates these sites, under glyphosate toxicity these sites are upregulated causing increased inflammation.[lvi] Adenosine receptors work in conjunction with GPCR sites to maintain homeostasis. Glyphosate changes the ratios of adenosine and guanine thus inducing activation of the adenosine receptor sites, inducing suppression of the immune system, triggering bronchospasm, increased heart rate, modifying calcium concentrations, etc.

v. Both the sympathetic and parasympathetic nervous systems are regulated by GPCR site pathways. These sites are responsible for control of many automatic functions of the body such as blood pressure, heart rate, and digestive processes. Glyphosate toxicity affects autonomic nervous system transmission, and dysregulation of the hypothalamic-pituitary-adrenal/-thyroid axes.

vi. Glyphosate disrupts homeostasis modulation (e.g., water balance) by affecting the GPCR sites in the pituitary.

vii. GPCR sites are involved in growth and metastasis of some types of tumors. Additionally, activation of the adenosine receptor sites encourages the growth of cancer cell lines. Macrophages that would normally be activated by their intramembrane GPCR receptors become obtuse and do not carry out their function of engulfing damaged cells.

viii. Glyphosate interrupts the functioning of the GPCR sites for hormones in the endocrine system resulting in infertility, thyroid, and metabolic issues.[lvii]

Glyphosate Creates High Serum Urate Levels:[lviii] The purine xanthine will be reduced to uric acid through normal metabolic processes. However, Glyphosate drives an excessive reduction to uric acid which can lead to uremic acidosis, then gout, when the uric acid levels are consistently high. Normally uric acid will pass out in the urine, however in high amounts, blood serum levels escalate and the uric acid either settles into joints in the form of gout, serves to leech calcium from the bones resulting in kidney stones, or produces system wide urticarial conditions such as hives.

Glyphosate, Vaccines, Retroviruses, Adenosine Receptor Sites, G-Protein Coupled Receptor Sites, Antibiotics, Inflammation, Heavy Metals the Immune System, and Autism:[lix] Vaccines are incubated on gelatin procured from the collagen of animals that have been raised on glyphosate sprayed food (glyphosate is stored in collagen). This means that in addition to giving an immunologically stimulating agent in a vaccine (viral or bacterial antigen) and the added aluminum adjuvants, used to further excite inflammatory antibody production, a glyphosate compounded chronic state of inflammation ensues.[lx]

We must also remember that inactivated (vaccine strain) verses live (wild) versions of viral or bacterial pathogens have the opposite effect on their organ of infinity. Childhood wild virus infectious diseases are meant to be contracted in childhood to strengthen the immune system towards an adaptive response designed for greater survivability.[lxi]

Conversely, when these attenuated (inactivated) viral strains are injected (such as the inactivated polio vaccine (IPV)), rather than touching on the mucosal membranes of the intestine, in the instance of the polio antigen, in combination with the vaccine adjuvants, serves to negatively upregulate zonulin (haptoglobin). Zonulin is a hormone excreted from the cells of the intestinal lining whose purpose is to maintain the integrity of the tight junctions in that intestinal lining.[lxii] When upregulated zonulin opens the tight junctions. IPV thus, opens the door for multiple antigens, proteins, and other inflammatory agents to enter the submucosa, circulatory system and ultimately the nervous system. The result of which is systemic inflammation. Conversely, oral polio vaccine (OPV) given at birth serves to facilitate the critical regulation of the tight junctions at the outset of life and long-term improved immune system function towards a variety of other diseases throughout life.[lxiii]

Glyphosate encourages the system to remain in a hyper-elevated state of inflammation through a number of interactions in addition to those afore mentioned:

i. Through a glyphosate driven deficiency of glycine for the glycine dependent glutamate receptors in the brain, promotes excess extracellular glutamate and a deficiency of GABA. This drives cerebral excitation, inflammation, and autistic expression.
ii. Glyphosate driven activation of the adenosine receptor sites suppresses the immune system's ability to develop the appropriate macrophage response needed to neutralize the newly injected bacterial or viral particles. This state of suppression elevates eosinophil and neutrophil counts, and mast cell degranulation resulting in increased allergic asthma and eczema.
iii. Glyphosate driven excess adenosine leads to suppression of zinc dependent adenosine deaminase (ADA) controlled RNA gene editing process. Some of the infectious agents in vaccines are RNA retroviruses (will upload into the hosts DNA to be replicated). With the immune system suppressed, co-infections with RNA retroviruses are transactivated which can effect further gene mutation.[lxiv] Associated retroviruses are Hepatitis

B, Human immunodeficiency virus (HIV), human T cell leukemia virus, and xenotropic murine leukemia virus (XMRV). (On a side note XMRV was found to have contaminated the inactivated polio vaccines (IPV) and compounds auto-immune dysregulation[lxv]).

iv. Immune system suppression also leads to activation of RNA viruses such as polio virus or herpes viruses. After their initial active stage, they will remain latent in the body only to become active when the immune system is suppressed or over taxed by other viruses: Herpes simplex, Chickenpox, EBV, Cytomegalovirus, etc.

v. This same suppression of the gene editing process affects the degradation of RNA viruses. These viruses also have a high mutation rate and can become incorporated into the DNA and modify gene expression. This quality of RNA viruses has enabled the science of GMO, by the insertion of RNA viruses into the DNA, and is unitized for all genetic modification of plants to make them disease resistant. The use of RNA viruses in vaccines has unwittingly modified gene expression in humans and rather than making them immune to the target disease, have rendered them in a greater state of ill-health as the viruses subject their functionality onto the cells of their organ of affinity. Human RNA viruses include:

   - Rotavirus, polio, and other enteroviruses (affecting zonulin (haptoglobin)and the regulation of the tight junctions in the intestines).
   - Ebola hemorrhagic fever, West Nile fever, Dengue, Yellow fever, and Zika* (affecting calcium and phosphorus in the bones, immune system and the liver with the blood clotting) mechanism.
   - Hepatitis C (affecting the liver).
   - SARS, common cold, influenza (affecting the respiratory and immune system).
   - Measles, Mumps and Rubella (affecting myelin in the brain, skin or intestinal lining, meninges, or glandular system respectively (gonads and breasts). The RNA viral strains in the MMR vaccine given to an individual with glyphosate toxicity will remain perpetually active causing inflammation

in their organs of affinity and will enter the DNA to modify gene expression.

- *Zika virus does not cause microcephaly. Reports show that those infants in Brazil born with microcephaly were born in areas heavily sprayed with the insecticide pyriproxyfen and this is the cause of the microcephaly. [lxvi] Contraction of Zika during pregnancy (when the antibody function of the immune system is naturally suppressed) may exacerbate the condition but the insecticide neurotoxin aimed at reducing mosquito populations is the root cause. Normal pathogenesis of Zika virus does not include a neurological affinity but transactivation of this virus by insecticides will compound the deleterious effects of the insecticide in the neurological system.

vi. The failure of the immune systems' ability to suppress the expression of these retroviruses results in aberrant immunological regulation, neurotransmitter ratios, and gene expression.[lxvii]

vii. The additional effect of the antibiotics used to suppress the macrophage directed elimination process that results in 'middle ear infections' leads to further gut biome dysbiosis, that is already dysregulated by glyphosate. This compounds the effects of the immunological and neuro-developmental delays previously discussed.[lxviii,lxix]

viii. Glyphosate driven interference of DNA coding for the digestive enzyme pepsin results in an inability to digest the gliadins in gluten which leads to inflammation in the intestinal lining. As a result, gluten and other toxins pass through the intestinal lining to the general circulation forcing an immune system response to the gluten.[lxx]

ix. Glyphosate compounds the toxicity of mercury (thimerosal, found in vaccines) by upregulating the pathological bacteria *Desulfovibrio,* which converts mercury to methylmercury which is far more toxic.[lxxi] In the face of glyphosate an individual with previous heavy metal toxicity will become that much more toxic as the leached mercury converts to methylmercury.

x. Glyphosate synergistically exaggerates the inflammatory response from the aluminum adjuvants added to vaccines compounding immune system inflammation.[lxxii]

xi. Vaccines disrupt the normal copper/zinc ratios in the brain. This is further compounded to the glyphosate driven copper excess and zinc deficiency. The copper/zinc ratio in is vital for DNA regulation in epigenetics, adenosine suppression of immunological expression, and acetylcholine activity and receptor site functionality. All of this increase the effect of autistic expression.[lxxiii]

xii. Interruption in neurotransmitter production in the gut and neurotransmitter regulation by glycine dependent receptor sites in the brain leads to a host of neurologic dysregulation patterns of expression.

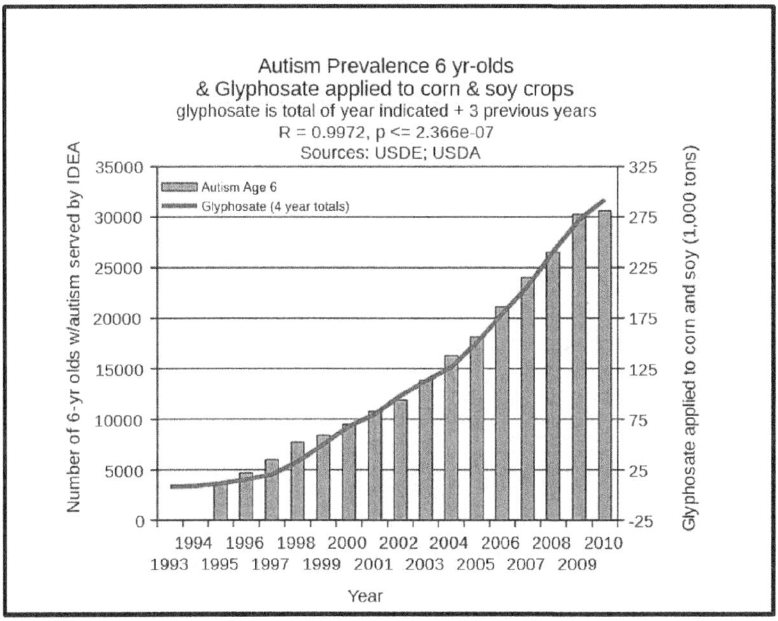

Comments: It is not a wonder why there is a proliferation in autism, pervasive developmental delays, depression, violence, and a host of other conditions of auto-dysregulation arising in today's children.[lxxiv,lxxv] Immune system function is coded by the DNA and is thus created by the blueprint of the **Generating-Organizing-Delivering/Destroying system**. Manmade environmental toxins that tinker with this basic code of life have corrupted its functionality and the health of the children suffers. These children will grow to be adults and demonstrate their suffering by a myriad of neurological and sociological pathologies. They are not to blame, rather, I hold those who have taken the charge of polluting the environment and those that are propagating and enforcing the vaccine and glyphosate agenda as responsible. The uptick in childhood developmental delays and autism (since 2000) corresponds directly to the expiration of Monsanto's patent on glyphosate and the corresponding global surge in its use.[lxxvi]

I also believe the consumer is equally responsible for creating the market that economically accepts this reality. We need to look at the shadow side of our disconnect: the fear and lack that makes us think we need to destroy the planet to feed ourselves, or at least to make a profit in the process; and the ignorance and gluttony that has left us weak to our ability to understand what we have caused in our lives and on this planet.

It is up to us to change the trajectory: for parents to become educated, for environmentalists, those that grow and manufacture food, and politicians alike, to face the facts that we are destroying the planet, and the human race, starting with children of the current generation, where 1 in 29 are diagnosed as autistic.[lxxvii]

As I compose this essay and begin to comprehend the ramifications of the disruption of the code of life, I am meditating on salvation from own glyphosate toxicity. Through researching and writing I have been searching for answers in my psyche from within the **Generating-Organizing Delivering/Destroying system** of this existence. I have been searching for answers in my own DNA about why it is I am here and what it is I can do.

As our DNA unfolds, we experience time, and as it unfolds, life and challenges come towards us. It is through the Rhodopsin-Like receptors in the organs of our chakric system we sense the external circumstances of life, the natural world we live in, and the people we are in connection with. These receptors, by design, when functional and clear, allow us to physically experience beauty and the bliss in the unified field. We become the pure expression and beauty of the blueprint that created this existence. When these receptors are blocked, polluted, and inoperable, then we experience separation from the field and suffer in the pain of that separation.

What I am explaining here is not a theoretical construct, but rather am using words to describe an experience of life that many including myself have attained. In my own life I have experienced that the closer to nature I come in my mind and body, no longer am I a servant to my ego-based desires or the mental constructs of my delusions. Rather, all I am and have become is a pure expression of that one system; viz GOD.

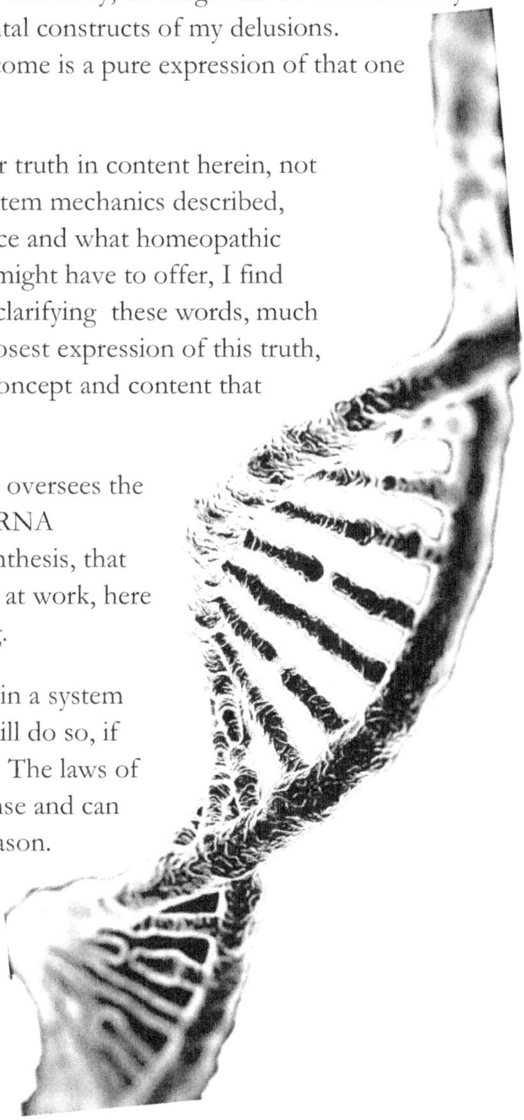

Accordingly, in my search for truth in content herein, not only of the science of the system mechanics described, but also in my life's experience and what homeopathic remedies and detoxification might have to offer, I find myself editing, refining, and clarifying these words, much like the DNA does, to the closest expression of this truth, to the purest experience of concept and content that comes through me.

This truth, like the force that oversees the editing of DNA replication, RNA transcription, and protein synthesis, that innate self-editing process, is at work, here in the words you are reading.

According to nature, we live in a system that is self-correcting, and will do so, if our ego steps out of the way. The laws of nature are basic common sense and can be understood by human reason.

These laws are objective and universal. If we were to apply our conscience as to how we interface with our being and the world, by nature, the results of those actions that are against nature will self-correct. If we settle into being, we become.

Rather, these days, what we see are individuals, nations, civilizations, and economic systems failing to recognize and regulate themselves. We have forgotten. There was a time when the human animal was sophisticated enough to articulate and actualize the complexities of the order in this life.
Now, through a number of destructive forces including the utilization of GMOs and glyphosate we have come to a macro- and micro- system failure including a disruption of the self-corrective editing force that aligns us with the force of the **Generating Organizing Delivering/ Destroying** aspects of our very own experience of beauty and truth.

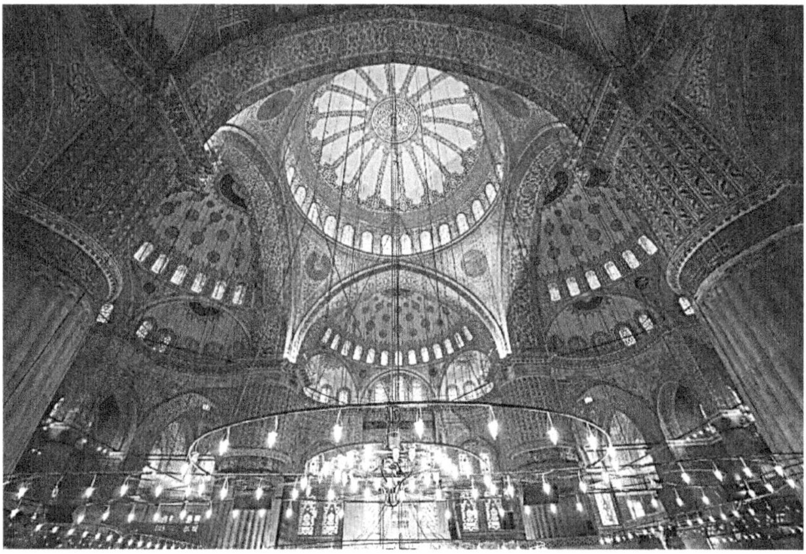

xxxvi Anthony Samsel, Stephanie Seneff. Glyphosate, pathways to modern diseases II: Celiac sprue and gluten intolerance. Interdiscip Toxicol. 2013 Dec. https://www.ncbi.nlm.nih.gov/pmc/articles/PMC3945755/.

xxxvii Tamsyn M Uren Webster, Eduarda M Santos. Global transcriptomic profiling demonstrates induction of oxidative stress and of compensatory cellular stress responses in brown trout exposed to glyphosate and Roundup. Jan 15, 2015. https://www.ncbi.nlm.nih.gov/pmc/articles/PMC4318436/.

xxxviii Marta Kwiatkowska, Jaromir Michałowicz, Paweł Jarosiewicz, Bożena Bukowska. The Impact of Glyphosate, Its Metabolites and Impurities on Viability, ATP Level and Morphological Changes in Human Peripheral Blood Mononuclear Cells. June 2016. https://www.researchgate.net/publication/304831091_The_Impact_of_Glyphosate_Its_Metabolites_and_Impurities_on_Viability_ATP_Level_and_Morphological_changes_in_Human_Peripheral_Blood_Mononuclear_Cells.

xxxix Christina Sarich. How Monsanto's Glyphosate Attacks our Core Cellular Functions. Global Research, January 20, 2016. https://www.globalresearch.ca/how-monsantos-glyphosate-attacks-our-core-cellular-functions/5502566.

xl Marta Kwiatkowska, Paweł Jarosiewicz, Jaromir Michałowicz, Maria Koter-Michalak, Bogumiła Huras, Bożena Bukowska. The Impact of Glyphosate, Its Metabolites and Impurities on Viability, ATP Level and Morphological changes in Human Peripheral Blood Mononuclear Cells. PLOS1. June 9, 2016. https://www.researchgate.net/publication/304831091_The_Impact_of_Glyphosate_Its_Metabolites_and_Impurities_on_Viability_ATP_Level_and_Morphological_changes_in_Human_Peripheral_Blood_Mononuclear_Cells.

xli Dan Dominissini, Sharon Moshitch-Moshkovitz, Ninette Amariglio, Gideon Rechavi. Adenosine-to-inosine RNA editing meets cancer. June 23, 2011. https://academic.oup.com/carcin/article/32/11/1569/2463282.

xlii Dipti Vijayan, Arabella Young, Michele W.L. Teng & Mark J. Smyth. Targeting immunosuppressive adenosine in cancer. 23 October. https://www.mendeley.com/catalogue/targeting-immunosuppressive-adenosine-cancer/.

xliii Scott H. Sicherer, MD, Mary E. Bollinger, DO, Michael S. Hershfield, MD, Hugh A. Sampson, MD, and Howard M. Lederman, MD, PhD. Food allergy in a patient with adenosine deaminase deficiency undergoing enzyme replacement with polyethylene glycol–modified adenosine deaminase. New York, N.Y., Baltimore, Md., and Durham, N.C. https://www.jacionline.org/article/S0091-6749(98)70408-7/pdf.

xliv Ibid.

xlv Sudhir Kumar, Marat Khodoun, Eric M. Kettleson, Christopher McKnight, Tiina Reponen, Sergey A. Grinshpun, and Atin Adhikari. Glyphosate–rich air samples induce IL–33, TSLP and generate IL–13 dependent airway inflammation. Toxicology. 2014 Nov 5; 0: 42–51. https://www.ncbi.nlm.nih.gov/pmc/articles/PMC4195794/.

xlvi T.D. Charlier (Rennes). Exposure to glyphosate and glyphosate-based herbicides during the peripartum period affects maternal behavior and maternal brain plasticity. Neuro France. 2017, Bordeaux, France. http://www.professionalabstracts.com/sn2017/programme-sn2017.pdf.

xlvii Judy A. Mikovits, Vincent C. Lombardi, Max A. Pfost, Kathryn S. Hagen, Francis W. Ruscetti. Detection of an infectious retrovirus, XMRV, in blood cells of patients with chronic fatigue syndrome. Virulence. 2010. Sep-Oct; 1(5): 386–390. https://www.ncbi.nlm.nih.gov/pmc/articles/PMC3073172/.

xlviii Dan Dominissini, Sharon Moshitch-Moshkovitz, Ninette Amariglio, Gideon Rechavi. Adenosine-to-inosine RNA editing meets cancer. Carcinogenesis, Volume 32, Issue 11, 1. November 2011, Pages 1569–1577. https://doi.org/10.1093/carcin/bgr124.

xlix Aparamita Pandeya, Medhamurthy Rudraiahb. Analysis of endocrine disruption effect of Roundup® in adrenal gland of male rats. Toxicology Reports. Volume 2, 2015, Pages 1075-1085. https://www.sciencedirect.com/science/article/pii/S221475001530041X.

l Mesnage R, Arno M, Costanzo M, Malatesta M, Séralini GE, Antoniou MN. Transcriptome profile analysis reflects rat liver and kidney damage following chronic ultra-low dose Roundup exposure. Environmental Health. 2015 Aug 25;14:70. https://www.ncbi.nlm.nih.gov/pubmed/26302742.

li DaianeCattani, Vera Lúciade, Liz Oliveira, CavalliCarla, EliseHeinz Rieg, Juliana Tonietto, Domingues Tharine Dal-Cim, Carla Inês, TascaFátima, ReginaMena, Barreto Silva, Ariane Zamoner. Mechanisms underlying the neurotoxicity induced by glyphosate-based herbicide in immature rat hippocampus: Involvement of glutamate excitotoxicity. Toxicology Volume 320, 5 June 2014, Pages 34-45. https://www.sciencedirect.com/science/article/pii/S0300483X14000493.

lii Seneff, Stephanie, Glyphosate+ Aluminum+ Mercury + Glutamate = Autism. AutismOne Media. June 1, 2018. https://www.youtube.com/watch?v=OL9mr599hb0.

liii Anthony Samsel, Stephanie Seneff. Glyphosate, pathways to modern diseases II: Celiac sprue and gluten intolerance. Interdiscip Toxicol. 2013 Dec. https://www.ncbi.nlm.nih.gov/pmc/articles/PMC3945755/.

liv Ibid.

lv Tamsyn M Uren Webster, Eduarda M Santos. Global transcriptomic profiling demonstrates induction of oxidative stress and of compensatory cellular stress responses in brown trout exposed to glyphosate and Roundup. BMC Genomics. 2015; 16(1): 32. https://www.ncbi.nlm.nih.gov/pmc/articles/PMC4318436/.

lvi Adhikari, Atin. TLR Ligand and Pesticide Exposure in Farms: Role in Atopic Immune Responses. NIH. University of Cincinnati, Cincinnati, OH, United States. http://grantome.com/grant/NIH/R21-ES017316-01A1.

lvii de Souza JS, Kizys MM, da Conceição RR, Glebocki G, Romano RM, Ortiga-Carvalho TM, Giannocco G, da Silva ID, Dias da Silva MR, Romano MA, Chiamolera MI. Perinatal exposure to glyphosate-based herbicide alters the thyrotrophic axis and causes thyroid hormone homeostasis imbalance in male rats. Toxicology. 2017 Feb 15;377:25-35. https://www.ncbi.nlm.nih.gov/pubmed/27916585.

lviii Stephanie Seneff, Laura F Orlando. Is Glyphosate a Key Factor in Mesoamerican Nephropathy? Journal of Environmental & Analytical Toxicology. 2018, 8:1.

lix John Slatterya, Derrick F. MacFabe, Stephen G. Kahlera, and Richard E. Fryea. Enteric Ecosystem Disruption in ASD. Current Pharmaceutical Design. Volume 22, Issue 40. 2016. https://www.ncbi.nlm.nih.gov/pubmed/27592717.

lx Birch, Kate. Vaccine Free Prevention and Treatment of Infectious Disease with Homeopathy. Create Space. USA. 2011.

lxi Birch, Kate. Whatcott, Cilla. The Solution ~ Homeoprophylaxis: The Vaccine Alternative. Create space, USA. 2011.

lxii Alessio Fasano. Zonulin, regulation of tight junctions, and autoimmune diseases. Ann N Y Acad Sci. 2012 Jul; 1258(1): 25–33. https://www.ncbi.nlm.nih.gov/pmc/articles/PMC3384703/.

lxiii Christine Stabell Benn. How vaccines train the immune system in ways no one expected. TEDxAarhus. https://www.youtube.com/watch?v=_d8PNlXHJ48.

lxiv Judy A. Mikovits, Vincent C. Lombardi, Max A. Pfost, Kathryn S. Hagen, Francis W. Ruscetti. Detection of an infectious retrovirus, XMRV, in blood cells of patients with chronic fatigue syndrome. Virulence. 2010. Sep-Oct; 1(5): 386–390. https://www.ncbi.nlm.nih.gov/pmc/articles/PMC3073172/.

lxv Ibid.

lxvi Is Zika the real cause of microcephaly in Brazil? New study raises questions. 10/09/2016. Health, News. https://inhabitat.com/is-zika-the-real-cause-of-microcephaly-in-brazil-new-study-raises-questions/.

lxvii Ibid.

lxviii T.D. Charlier (Rennes). Exposure to glyphosate and glyphosate-based herbicides during the peripartum period affects maternal behavior and maternal brain plasticity. Neuro France. 2017, Bordeaux, France. https://www.ncbi.nlm.nih.gov/pubmed/27592717.

lxix Bilbo SD, Nevison CD, Parker W. A model for the induction of autism in the ecosystem of the human body: the anatomy of a modern pandemic? Microb Ecol Health Dis, 2015; 26: 26253. https://www.ncbi.nlm.nih.gov/pubmed/25634608.

lxx Seneff, S. Glyphosate + aluminum + mercury + glutamate = autism. AutismOne Media. June 1, 2018. https://www.youtube.com/watch?v=OL9mr599hb0.

lxxi Ibid.

lxxii Ibid.

lxxiii Fatemeh Sayehmiri, MSc, Nasim Babaknejad, MSc, Somayeh Bahrami, MSc, Kourosh Sayehmiri, PhD, Mojtaba Darabi, MD ,1 and Mostafa Rezaei-Tavirani, PhD. Zn/Cu Levels in the Field of Autism Disorders: A Systematic Review and Meta-analysis. Iran J Child Neurol. 2015 Autumn; 9(4): 1–9. https://www.ncbi.nlm.nih.gov/pmc/articles/PMC4670971/.

lxxiv John Slatterya, Derrick F. MacFabe, Stephen G. Kahlera, and Richard E. Fryea. Enteric Ecosystem Disruption in ASD. Current Pharmaceutical Design. Volume 22, Issue 40. 2016. https://www.ncbi.nlm.nih.gov/pubmed/27592717.

lxxv Coulter, Harris, Fisher, Barbara, Loe. A Shot in the Dark: Why the P in the DPT may be hazardous to your child's health. Avery Trade. 1991.

lxxvi Dr. Nancy Swanson. The Autism Epidemic: Data show correlations between increase in neurological diseases and GMOs. 4/6/2013.

http://myfoodstuff.net/application/files/1514/9046/2512/GMO-6_neurological_disease.pdf.

lxxvii Weiler, James Lyons. US CDC: Autism Rate At Least 1 in 29 (DSM-5), 1 in 59 (DSM-IV). Cures. April 27, 2018. https://jameslyonsweiler.com/2018/04/27/us-cdc-autism-rate-at-least-1-in-29-dsm-v-1-in-59-dsm-iv/.

4. Glyphosate and Protein Structure

1. DNA transcribes RNA. RNA synthesizes proteins from free floating amino acids (basic nitrogen contain building blocks) on the endoplasmic reticulum in a cell's interior.
2. Strands of proteins form primary, secondary, tertiary, and quaternary bonds as the protein complexes are formed. We need enzymes to digest the protein we eat, and we need enzymes to make our structural and functional proteins. Enzymes are also proteins.
3. All proteins are assembled from amino acids sourced from the food we eat or are synthesized in our cells. There are 22 amino acids, 13 of which are essential to our diet (must be sourced outside of our body). The remaining 9 can be synthesized within our cells.
4. Glycine is a non-essential amino acid created in our body but also sourced from meat, fish, eggs, and legumes.
5. DNA replication and RNA transcription and protein synthesis are critically stimulated, regulated, and moderated by glycine dependent purines, pyrimidines, and enzymes.
6. Normal bacteria in the intestines synthesize the amino acid tryptophan, and phenylalanine, the precursor for tyrosine. These in turn form the bases for the monoamine neurotransmitters dopamine, norepinephrine, and epinephrine (adrenaline).
7. Tyrosine is also the precursor to trypsin, the enzyme needed to digest wheat gluten. The thyroid hormones, triiodothyronine (T3) and thyroxine (T4), made in the colloid of the thyroid, are also derived from tyrosine.
8. In a primary protein sequence, amino acids are linked together by peptide bonds. Trypsin is needed to hydrolyze the bonds between glycine and lysine or arginine.
9. Secondary and tertiary protein bonds are weak hydrogen bonds and are functional bonds, which means they open and close based on instructions from the environment: e.g. heating and cooling, acid/base conditions or other enzymes. The secondary bond structure, that of a helix shape, e.g. the two nucleotide chains in DNA, are what enables the DNA to zip open and close, turn on

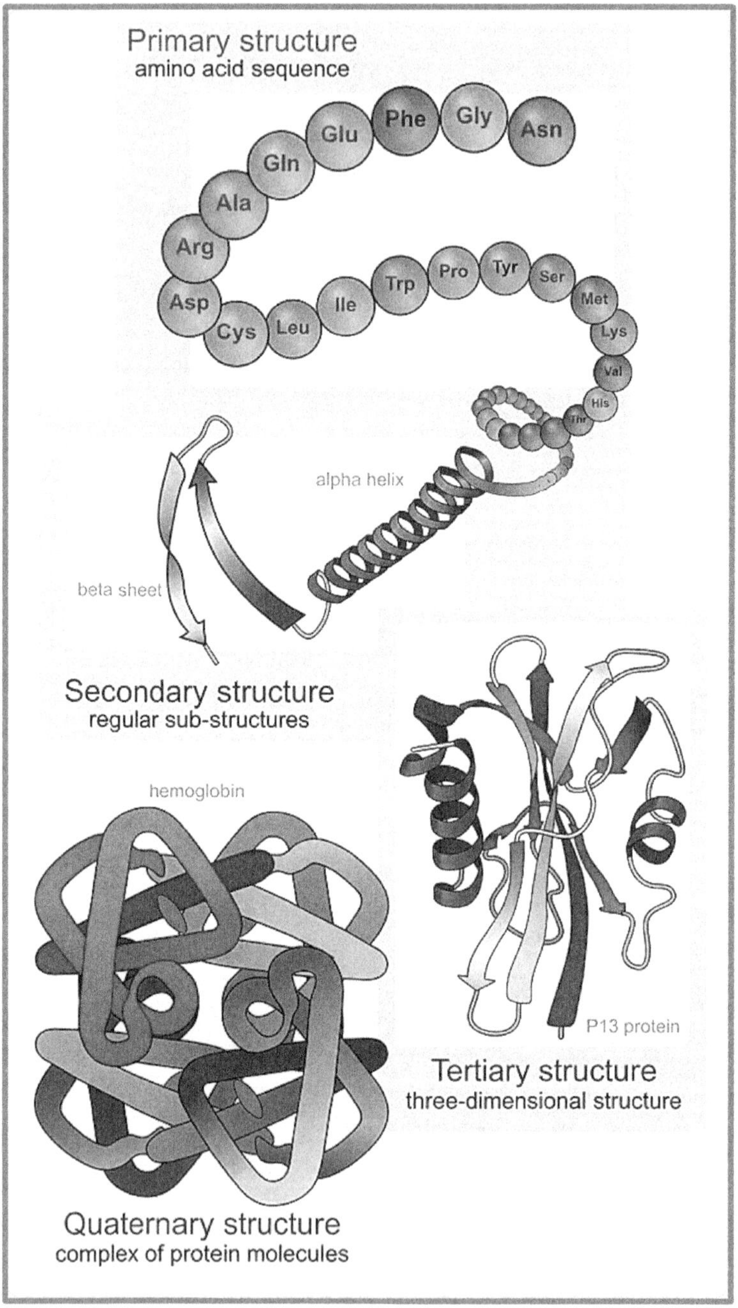
Primary structure
amino acid sequence
Phe
Gly
Asn
Glu
Gln
Ala
Arg
Asp
Cys
Leu
Ile
Trp
Pro
Tyr
Ser
Met
Lys
Val
His
Thr
alpha helix
beta sheet
Secondary structure
regular sub-structures
hemoglobin
P13 protein
Tertiary structure
three-dimensional structure
Quaternary structure
complex of protein molecules

and off genes and stimulate or suppress RNA transcription and protein synthesis.

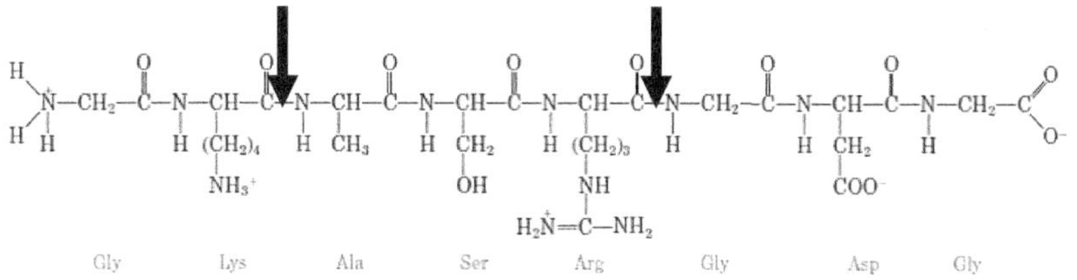

The enzyme trypsin catalyzes the hydrolysis of the amino acid peptide bond at the points marked with an arrow, (the carboxyl side of lysine or arginine).

10. Tertiary bonds between adjacent amino acids in enzymes allow them to work (act as cleavers) in liberating functional subunit proteins needed for other reactions. G-protein coupled receptors (GPCRs) sites are functional by enzymatic action on these tertiary bonds in the receptor.
11. Quaternary structure is established by disulfide bonds between the sulfur units of amino acids. Methionine, cysteine, homocysteine, and taurine are amino acids containing sulfur. These bonds need the enzyme sulfite oxidase, which is molybdenum dependent to be functional.
12. Through a series of enzymatic pathways, fortified with vitamins and minerals, glycine dependent proteins and enzymes are formed and converted to intermediaries that regulate, detox, and contribute to multiple metabolic functions in the cells.

    Histamine is a hydrophilic (water attracting = tissue swelling) amine derived protein from the decarboxylation of the amino acid histidine. It is an immune agent and a neurotransmitter. It is produced in basophils and mast cells of the immune system located in the fascia and on the mucous membranes of the nose, mouth, blood vessels, and intestinal lining and is part of the immune response triggered by infectious agents. In the brain it acts as a neurotransmitter that regulates a variety of physiological functions including sleep-wake cycles, appetite, memory, and the stress response. It is synthesized in the mast cells long with tryptase. Histamine is also formed by bacteria in some foods. If we have developed IgE antibodies to these foods, the mast cell membranes are activated by these antigens. and can produce localized inflammation, itching, and hives. Histamine also regulates blood vasodilation, immune response, neurotransmitter production, and circadian rhythms. Histamine is methylated by the enzymes histamine-N-methyltransferase (in the brain) and oxidized by diamine oxidase (DAO) (rest of the body).

15. Histamine-N-methyltransferase catalyzes the methylation of histamine in the presence of S-adenosylmethionine (SAM) (SAMe) which is formed in the liver but by also *E. coli* bacteria. Histamine-N-methyltransferase (HNMT) is produced by the Astroglia cells in the brain and reduces histamine found in the brain as diamine oxidase (DAO) is not produced there and cannot cross the blood brain barrier.
16. Methionine is an essential amino acid derived from nuts, meat, fish, eggs, dairy, and *Bifidobacteria.* In the MTHFR gene regulated methylation cycle methionine is a precursor to homocysteine, then cysteine which then, combined with glycine, forms glutathione. In MTHFR gene mutations this folate dependent glutathione methylation pathway is disrupted.

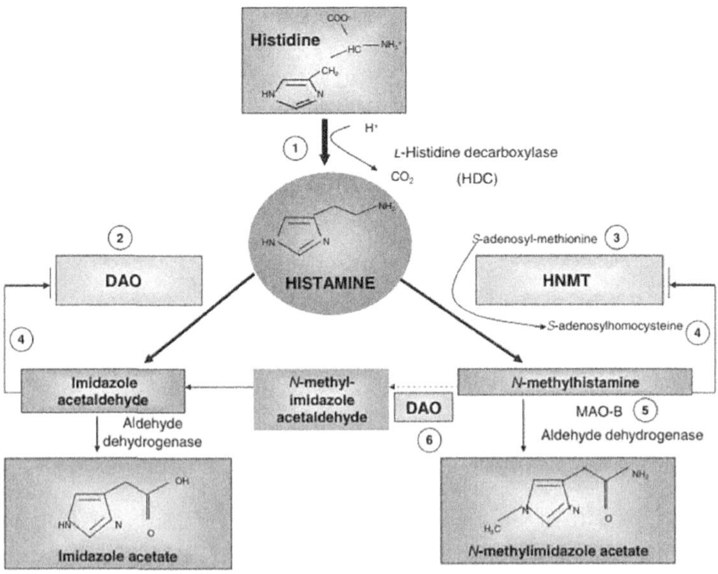

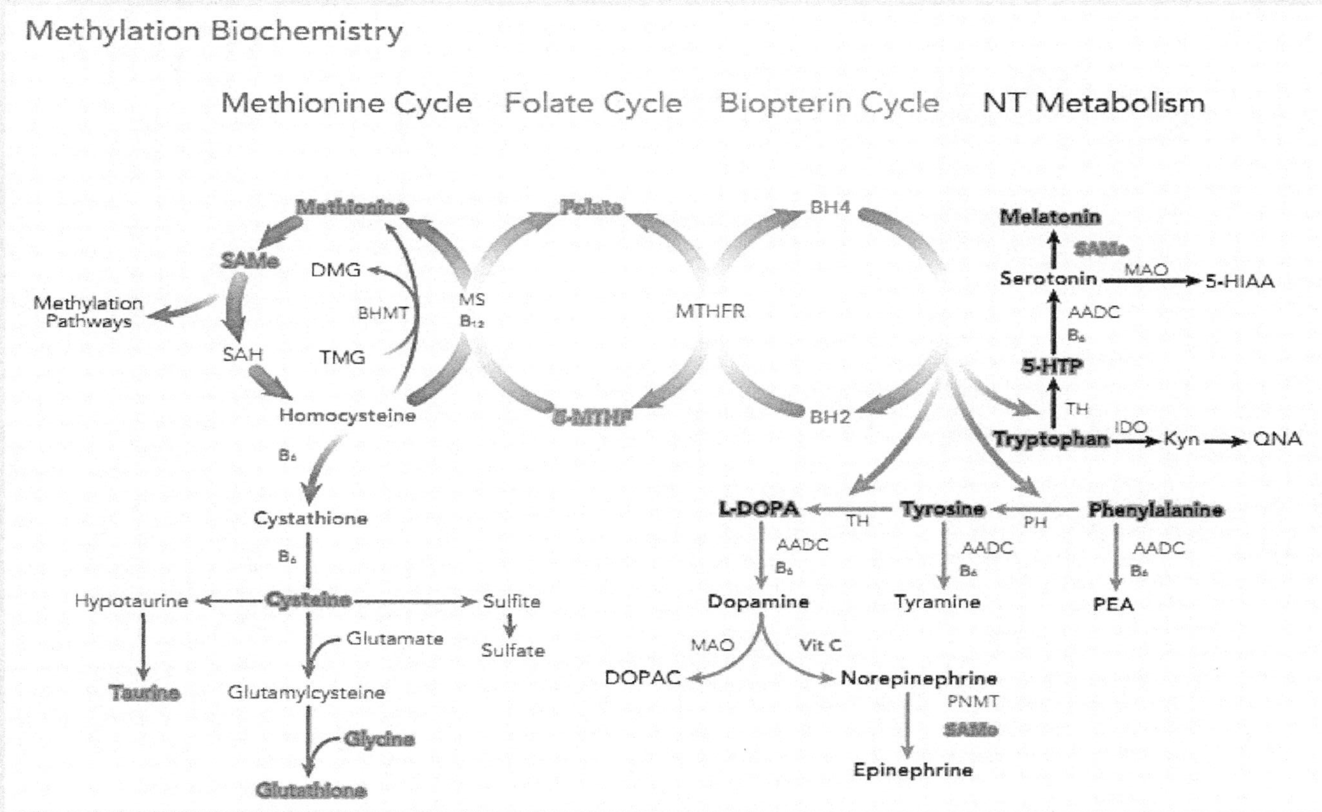
Methylation Biochemistry
Methionine Cycle
Folate Cycle
Biopterin Cycle
NT Metabolism
Methionine
SAMe
DMG
Methylation Pathways
BHMT
MS
B12
SAH
TMG
Homocysteine
B6
Cystathione
B6
Hypotaurine
Cysteine
Sulfite
Sulfate
Glutamate
Taurine
Glutamylcysteine
Glycine
Glutathione
Folate
MTHFR
5-MTHF
BH4
BH2
Melatonin
SAMe
Serotonin
MAO
5-HIAA
AADC
B6
5-HTP
TH
Tryptophan
IDO
Kyn
QNA
L-DOPA
TH
Tyrosine
PH
Phenylalanine
AADC
B6
AADC
B6
AADC
B6
Dopamine
Tyramine
PEA
MAO
Vit C
DOPAC
Norepinephrine
PNMT
SAMe
Epinephrine

17. The vitamin pyridoxine (B6), another *Bifidobacteria* dependent vitamin, is necessary to convert homocysteine to cysteine which is easily oxidized and is used in many biological processes. It naturally binds to metals for chelation. Pyridoxine (B6) protects against depression, anxiety, insomnia, age-related cognitive decline, hypoglycemia, kidney stones, and the morning sickness of pregnancy.
18. Glutathione is a tripeptide derived from glutamic acid, cysteine, and glycine which are dependent on methionine as the substrate. Glutathione is a sulfur containing antioxidant that works to remove free radicals, inflammatory agents, and heavy metals from the body. Its functionality is due to the action of sulfite oxidase on its quaternary disulfide bonds. Insufficient sulfite oxidase leads to an inability to properly utilize glutathione which results in a body unable to break down toxins for elimination. Glutathione is also responsible to reduce oxidative stress which drives elevated histamine levels. Cobalamin (B12) and folate (B9) are needed to transsulphurate homocysteine to cysteine.
19. The folate (B9) cycle is also dependent upon methionine.

Glyphosate and Protein Structure:

i. Glyphosate supplants glycine in protein synthesis. Glycine is coded by the nucleotides G-C-C. While transcribing RNA in protein synthesis, glyphosate is inserted in all the places glycine is called for. This produces a protein with an extra methyl group that disrupts the ability of that protein to fold and/or function accordingly. If the enzymes needed for editing RNA and DNA are corrupted by glyphosate the instructions are improper and the proteins and enzymes created will malfunction.[lxxviii]
ii. Those enzymes that are glycine dependent will uptake glyphosate instead of glycine. If glyphosate stimulates defective editing of RNA protein synthesis then a host of issues will follow such as gene mutation, and dysfunctional proteins and enzymes.[lxxix]
iii. The bacteria in our intestines, supplant glyphosate for glycine in transcription of the enzyme EPSP synthase, necessary for the synthesis of the aromatic amino acids tryptophan, phenylalanine, and tyrosine. The first two of which are considered essential amino

acids, needing to come from food, or to be created by the bacteria living in our intestines.[lxxx]

iv. The antibiotic action of glyphosate on lacto-fermenting bacteria and subsequent tyrosine deficiencies, leads to deficiencies in trypsin, the enzyme necessary to digest wheat gluten and for thyroxine (T4) to triiodothyronine (T3) conversion. Gluten intolerance and thyroid disfunction will develop.[lxxxi]

v. Glyphosate drives glycine, cobalamin (B12), folate (B9), or sulfur deficiencies. This reduces glutathione levels leading to increased metabolic and heavy metal toxicity and dysregulation of the complex methylation pathway utilized to create glutathione, folate (B9), and neurotransmitters. MTHFR gene mutations compound this issue.[lxxxii]

vi. Glyphosate is a combination of glycine and an extra phosphate group. The presence of this extra phosphate interferes with and disrupts functionality of the secondary and tertiary bonds between proteins. Glyphosate incorporated into G-protein coupled receptors (GPCRs) sites disable them.[lxxxiii]

vii. Quaternary sulfur bonds need the enzyme sulfite oxidase, which is molybdenum dependent, to be functional. Glyphosate depletes molybdenum thus sulfite oxidase. Glutathione functionality is based upon sulfite oxidase.

viii. The entire methylation pathway of glutathione, folate (B9), biopterin and neurotransmitter metabolism is affected by glyphosate. [lxxxiv]

ix. Histamine production is regulated by genes. Glyphosate driven glycine dependent dysregulation of genetic expression leads to dysregulation of the normal feedback loops that keep histamine levels in check. Glyphosate also causes a reduction in diamine oxidase (DAO) (glycine dependent) allowing system wide inflammatory states to persist. Glyphosate may contribute to depletion of histamine-N-methyltransferase resulting in elevated histamine in the brain leading to increased wakefulness, aggressive behavior, hitting, biting, memory deficiencies, and neurological developmental delays: all symptoms that are consistent with autism.

x. Glyphosate inhibits CYP450 enzymes which raises histamine levels. Heparan sulfate is one such enzyme that reduces the amount of histamine being released from mast cells. Heparan is a proteoglycan, a large protein complex, consisting of mainly glycine, and found in the connective tissue (fascia) of the body. Glyphosate insertion when glycine is coded for, renders this enzyme defective. Deficiency in heparan sulfate leads to build up of histamines.[lxxxv]

xi. Glyphosate interrupts the *Bifidobacteria* dependent biosynthesis of the B vitamin pyridoxine (B6), that coverts homocysteine to cysteine in the glutathione methylation pathway.

xii. Glyphosate is responsible for insufficient glutathione due to the methionine deficiency from depletion of the bacteria that produce methionine.[lxxxvi]

---

lxxviii Seneff, S., Morley, W., Hadden, M.J., Michener, M.C. Does glyphosate acting as a glycine analogue contribute to ALS? Journal of. Bioinformatics Proteomics Rev. 2 (2016):1–21.

lxxix Ibid.

lxxx Todd Funke, Huijong Han, Martha L. Healy-Fried, Markus Fischer, and Ernst Schönbrunn. Molecular basis for the herbicide resistance of Roundup-Ready crops. Proceedings of the National Academy of Sciences of the United States of America. 2006 Aug 29; 103(35): 13010–13015. https://www.ncbi.nlm.nih.gov/pmc/articles/PMC1559744/.

lxxxi Anthony Samsel and Stephanie Seneff. Glyphosate, pathways to modern diseases II: Celiac sprue and gluten intolerance. Interdiscip Toxicol. 2013 Dec. https://www.ncbi.nlm.nih.gov/pmc/articles/PMC3945755/.

lxxxii Ibid.

lxxxiii Yassine Ait Bali, Saadia Ba-Mhamed, and Mohamed Bennis. Behavioral and Immunohistochemical Study of the Effects of Sub chronic and Chronic Exposure to Glyphosate in Mice. Frontiers in Behavioral Neuroscience. 2017; 11: 146. https://www.ncbi.nlm.nih.gov/pmc/articles/PMC5550406/.

lxxxiv Anthony Samsel and Stephanie Seneff. Glyphosate, pathways to modern diseases II: Celiac sprue and gluten intolerance. Interdiscip Toxicol. 2013 Dec. https://www.ncbi.nlm.nih.gov/pmc/articles/PMC3945755/.

lxxxv Stephanie Seneff. Sulfate Deficiency in Neurological Disease Following Aluminum and Glyphosate Exposure. June 2, 2015. https://people.csail.mit.edu/seneff/2015/SeneffJune2_2015.pdf.

lxxxvi Anthony Samsel and Stephanie Seneff. Glyphosate, pathways to modern diseases II: Celiac sprue and gluten intolerance. Interdiscip Toxicol. 2013 Dec. https://www.ncbi.nlm.nih.gov/pmc/articles/PMC3945755/.

5. Glyphosate, Sugar, and Fat Metabolism

Photosynthesis: A process by which plant cells harness the light energy of the sun into chemical energy through the Calvin cycle. In the plant cell mitochondria carbon dioxide (CO_2) and water (H_2O) are synthesized into glucose, liberating oxygen in the process. The energy for the process comes from the liberation of one phosphate group from adenosine triphosphate (ATP) reducing it to adenosine diphosphate (ADP). This is represented in the following equation. The precursor of glucose is glyceraldehyde-3-phosphate = G_3P.

$$3\ CO_2 + 6\ NADPH + 6\ H^+ + 9\ ATP \rightarrow (G3P) + 6\ NADP+ + 9\ ADP + 3\ H_2O + 8\ P_i$$

The sugars produced during carbon dioxide metabolism are carbon molecules (carbohydrates) that can be utilized for other metabolic reactions like the production of amino acids (carbon, hydrogen, oxygen, and nitrogen molecules) and lipids (carbon, hydrogen, and oxygen). These biproducts are used as the energy currency for other chemical reactions within the plant cells and serve as the food sources for other living creatures.

It is believed the first photosynthetic organisms evolved early in the evolutionary history of life and most likely used the reducing agents

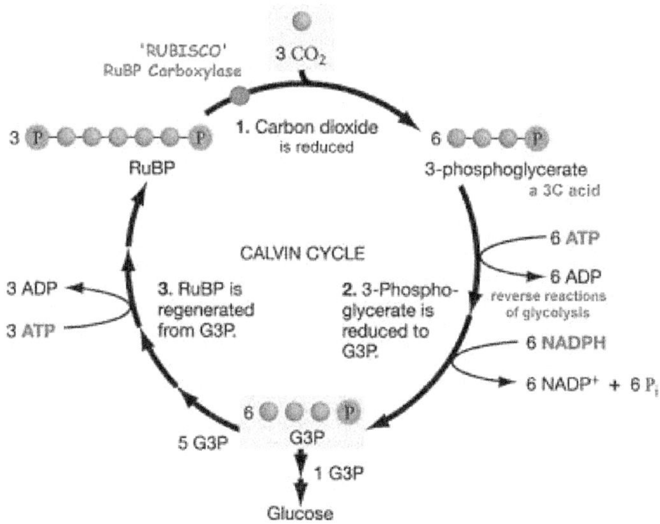

such as hydrogen or hydrogen sulfide, rather than water as sources of electrons. *Cyanobacteria* appeared later, and the excess oxygen they produced contributed directly to the oxygenation of the earth. This rendered the evolution of complex life possible through aerobic respiration (glycolysis). *Cyanobacteria* remain the main producers of oxygen on this earth and are critical to all marine ecosystems.

Aerobic Respiration: A metabolic reaction that takes place in the mitochondria of living organisms, in the presence of oxygen, where glucose (derived from plant or animal sources) and oxygen are converted back to carbon dioxide and water, producing the cellular energy units of ATP. Bacteria that inhabit the digestive systems of insects, reptiles, birds, and mammals produce the enzymes needed to metabolize sugars, proteins, and fats into ATP for all cellular functions. In the process CO_2 and H_2O are liberated. Mitochondria of more complex organisms complete this same process.

There are four steps to this process. Simple sugars (glucose) are metabolized to produce ATP with the enzymatic help of nicotinamide adenine dinucleotide (NAD^+) (contains the nucleotides nicotine and adenine). NAD^+ is a cofactor to functionality of the enzymes used in this and many other processes. Humans and other animals are carbon dioxide producers through the glycolysis process.

1. Glycolysis:
   - 2 ATPs + Glucose → 2 Pyruvic Acid + 4 Hydrogen (H^+) + 4 ATPs
2. Formation of Acetyl CoA (coenzyme A):
   - 2 Pyruvic Acid + 2 CoA → 2 Acetyl CoA + 2 Carbon Dioxide (CO_2)+ 2 H^+
3. Krebs Cycle (Citric acid cycle):
   - 2 Acetyl CoA + 3 O_2 → 6 H^+ + 4 CO_2+ 2 ATPs
4. Electron Transport System:
   - 12 H^+ + 3 O_2 → 6 Water (H_2O) + 32 ATPs

Overall Reaction:

- Glucose + 6 O_2 → 6 CO_2 + 6 H_2O + 36 ATPs

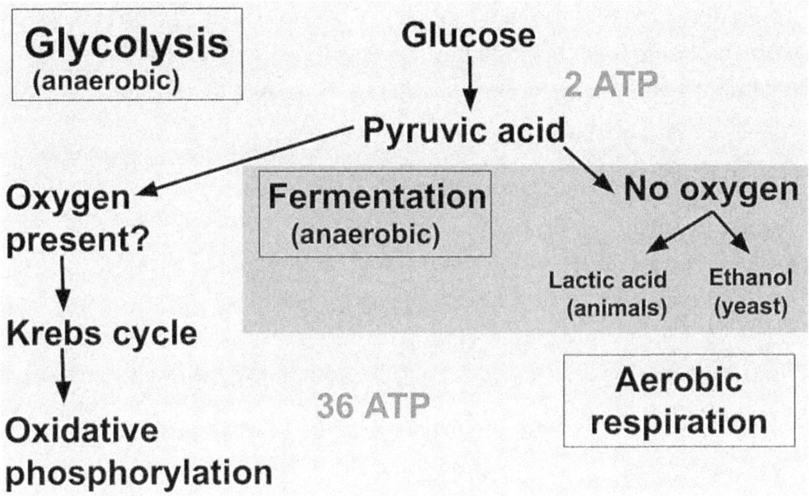

Anerobic Respiration: If insufficient oxygen is available in step 2, pyruvic acid is anaerobically fermented by lacto-fermenting bacteria to lactic acid instead of carbon dioxide and water, producing only two units of ATP. In wine making, the malic acid present in the fruit is converted to lactic acid by this same family of bacteria.

Bacteria also facilitate the anaerobic fermentation of fiber, fats (fatty acids), and glucose in cheese making, sourdough products, kombucha, and fermented vegetables (sauerkraut), etc.

Yeasts thrive in low oxygen environments and convert pyruvic acid to ethanol (alcohol). Yeasts facilitate the production of alcohol in wine and beer. In the human intestines yeast populations also produce ethanol which is marked by sweat or alcoholic smelling breath.

In the intestines, bacteria also metabolize fiber to produce the short-chain fatty acids (SCFAs) through acetyl CoA conversion (step 2). Here, fatty acids can be used as energy sources to build the protective mucous layers of the intestine, to enhance gut motility, and control the gene regulation of cellular proliferation and immune responses.

Pyruvic acid can also ferment to produce the amino acid alanine. Alanine is a simple non-essential amino acid in humans. Alanine, next to glycine, is one of the most widely used amino acids for protein construction and is involved in the recycling of tryptophan and the vitamin pyridoxine (B6). It also helps in the oxidation of glutamate to ammonia in the liver.

The mitochondria in muscle cells will metabolize sugars to produce energy through the Krebs cycle (step 3). Thus, in the presence of oxygen, lactic acid is not produced. With prolonged exercise, in muscles that are not used to exercising, reduced levels of oxygen drive lactic acid production resulting in pain and stiffness in the muscles. This lactic acid is sent to the liver to be metabolized through the Cori cycle (lactic acid cycle).

When oxygen supply is insufficient, typically during intense muscular activity, energy (ATP) for continued exertion must be produced through anaerobic metabolism (lactic acid fermentation). In this instance pyruvic acid converts directly to lactate (lactic acid + H+) by lactate dehydrogenase. Nicotinamide adenine dinucleotide (NAD^+) is synthesized from the amino acids tryptophan and aspartic acid. Lactic acid fermentation, towards the creation of lactate with lactate dehydrogenase (LD), serves to maintain NAD^+ concentrations so that additional glycolysis reactions can occur. During fasting this process is enhanced. Thus, fasting and increasing oxygen levels lowers lactic acid levels, subsequently increasing NAD^+.

Lactic acidosis: An excess of lactic acid or lactate occurs when the system becomes excessively acidic (low pH). It occurs in conditions of oxygen starvation (excessive exercise, stroke like conditions, prolonged fevers, sepsis, shock, diabetes, mitochondrial encephalopathy, or medication), genetic metabolism disorders, or an NAD^+ dependent enzyme deficiency forcing insufficient lactic acid fermentation. Either pyruvate dehydrogenase (step 2: production of Acetyl CoA), or pyruvate carboxylase (needed in step 3: Krebs cycle), depending.

Lactic acidosis is marked by an excess of hydrogen ions as a result of pyruvic acid converting directly to $lactate^-$ and H^+, rather than lactic acid, by bypassing the normally pH buffered lactic acid – lactate conversion system. When the system is saturated with lactic acid, as in low oxygen systems (prolonged fever or exercise), the extra hydrogen atoms create an acidic system: an acidic system has a high number of free hydrogen (H^+) atoms (low pH). Vaginal pH needs to be acidic. It is populated with *Lactobacillus* which produces lactic acid that maintains this acidity. On the other hand, systemic acidity and elevated lactic acid can lead to a myriad of problems.

Lactic acidosis can present as nausea, vomiting, white tongue, labored and deep breathing, with generalized weakness. Some forms of lactic acidosis are caused by mitochondrial disease. In severe infections (whereby the fever has used up all the oxygen in the blood) it may cause an increased risk of death. Lactic acidosis and elevated histamine can lead to cerebral inflammation, developmental delays, autism, and changes in mood and behavior.

Fats: Saturated, and poly- or mono-saturated, depending on the number of hydrogen atoms in the chemical structure, are composed of fatty acid building blocks. Saturated fats, mostly from animal sources are essential in the creation of the 'good' cholesterol which is the precursor for steroid hormones and used throughout the body for a myriad of essential functions. Cholesterol is also the precursor for bile acids, which are synthesized by the liver then transported to the gut, where they aid in the digestion of dietary fat. Saturated fats produce low-density lipoproteins (LDLs) which can lead to high 'bad' cholesterol levels and clogging of the cardiovascular system.

Poly-unsaturated fats are sourced from vegetable (corn, soybean, safflower, and sunflower) and fish oils. These high-density lipoproteins (HDLs) can serve to lower "bad' cholesterol and LDLs, however they will also lower the levels of "good" cholesterol needed for bile acid and hormone creation.

Mono-unsaturated fats such as oils derived from nuts, olive oil, peanut, and canola oil reduce LDL levels without reducing the beneficial cholesterol.

Trans-fats, oils made from poly-unsaturated fats that have been hydrogenated, where extra hydrogen molecules had been added to harden and stabilize the fat, render useless any positive benefit of the unsaturated fat. Trans-fats, widely produced industrially from vegetable fats, are found in margarine, snack foods, packaged baked goods, and for frying fast food. Trans-fats cause an increased risk of coronary artery disease, a leading cause of death in western nations.

Glyphosate and Sugar Metabolism:

i. Glyphosate's primary target is the shikimate-acid pathway in bacteria and plant cells. The shikimate-acid pathway is utilized to create ATP for all cellular functions in bacteria.[lxxxvii]
ii. Due to Glyphosate verses glycine assimilation nucleotide formation and DNA and RNA replication which require glycine is disrupted.[lxxxviii] Malfunctioning RNA cannot code normal enzyme production and those enzymes dependent on glycine will not function.[lxxxix] This disrupts mitochondrial function and ATP production.[xc, xci] ATP is needed in photosynthesis to produce carbohydrates.
iii. Glyphosate preferentially kills the lacto fermenting bacteria that convert sugars to carbon dioxide, water and ATP.[xcii]

Glyphosate and Fat Metabolism:

i. While glyphosate is water soluble and not found in vegetable oils, it is present in all the GMO wheat and corn fed to commercially-raised livestock. The hybridization of wheat to increase gluten content in turn increased the fat content of the meat produced. This higher level of fat, when consumed by humans, increases the HDLs and resultant 'bad' cholesterol levels and lowers the production of bile acids necessary to metabolize this form of fat. The result of which is constipation and the formation of calcified cholesterol (plaque) on the arterial walls.[xciii]
ii. Glyphosate interferes with the shikimate-acid pathway of all lacto-fermenting bacteria; it is disturbed due to interference in the creation of EPSP synthase and is a chelator of iron. Iron and EPSP synthase are necessary for the synthesis of cytochrome P450-Enzymes. These are heme-dependent enzymes needed in the liver to create bile acids and bile salts for fat emulsification and metabolism.[xciv]

lxxxvii Todd Funke, Huijong Han, Martha L. Healy-Fried, Markus Fischer, and Ernst Schönbrunn. Molecular basis for the herbicide resistance of Roundup-Ready crops. Proceedings of the National Academy of Sciences of the United States of America. 2006 Aug 29; 103(35): 13010–13015. https://www.ncbi.nlm.nih.gov/pmc/articles/PMC1559744/.

lxxxviii Seneff, S., Morley, W., Hadden, M.J., Michener, M.C. Does glyphosate acting as a glycine analogue contribute to ALS? Journal of. Bioinformatics Proteomics Rev. 2 (2016):1–21.

lxxxix Yassine Ait Bali, Saadia Ba-Mhamed, and Mohamed Bennis. Behavioral and Immunohistochemical Study of the Effects of Sub chronic and Chronic Exposure to Glyphosate in Mice. Frontiers in Behavioral Neuroscience. 2017; 11: 146. https://www.ncbi.nlm.nih.gov/pmc/articles/PMC5550406/.

xc Marta Kwiatkowska, Jaromir Michałowicz, Paweł Jarosiewicz, Bożena Bukowska. The Impact of Glyphosate, Its Metabolites and Impurities on Viability, ATP Level and Morphological Changes in Human Peripheral Blood Mononuclear Cells. June 2016. https://www.researchgate.net/publication/304831091_The_Impact_of_Glyphosate_Its_Metabolites_and_Impurities_on_Viability_ATP_Level_and_Morphological_changes_in_Human_Peripheral_Blood_Mononuclear_Cells.

xci Anthony Samsel and Stephanie Seneff. Glyphosate, pathways to modern diseases II: Celiac sprue and gluten intolerance. Interdiscip Toxicol. 2013 Dec. https://www.ncbi.nlm.nih.gov/pmc/articles/PMC3945755/.

xcii Seneff, Stephanie. Glyphosate+ Aluminum+ Mercury + Glutamate= Autism. AutismOne Media. June 1, 2018. https://www.youtube.com/watch?v=OL9mr599hb0.

xciii Greg Lardy, John Dhuyvetter. Feeding Wheat to Beef Cattle. NDSU, North Central Research Extension Center, Minot. https://www.ag.ndsu.edu/publications/livestock/feeding-wheat-to-beef-cattle.

xciv Seneff, Stephanie. Glyphosate+ Aluminum+ Mercury + Glutamate= Autism. AutismOne Media. June 1, 2018. https://www.youtube.com/watch?v=OL9mr599hb0.

6. Glyphosate and the Biome

The vital force, consciousness, thought forms, metabolic processes, neurotransmitter production, and the endocrine and immunological functions of the human animal are a direct result of the functioning and vitality of the natural biome and its interface with his intestinal lining. The biome includes the bacteria that cover the surface of our bodies and all mucous membranes.

The most dominant bacterial phyla in the human biome belong to the genera *Bacteroides*, *Clostridia*, *Faecalibacterium*, *Eubacterium*, *Peptococcus*, *Peptostreptococcus*,. *Staphylococcus*, and *Bifidobacteria*. Other genera, such as *Eschericha* (*E. coli*) and *Lactobacillus* are present to a lesser extent. Species from the genus Bacteroides alone constitute about 30% of all bacteria in the gut, suggesting that this genus is especially important in the functioning of the individual. In health, our biome has an innate vitality that connects us to the truth of our existence in nature: our vitality is reflective of the natural vitality of the biome within us. When healthy bacteria are displaced, pathological bacteria and *Candida* multiply.

The biome is responsible for facilitating multiple functions including, but not limited to, metabolism and digestive processes, hormonal regulation, immune system function, neurotransmitter production and regulation, blood clotting, and normal childhood development. Bacteria on the skin enable it to heal and prevents opportunistic infections from invasive species. The gut flora itself appears to function like an endocrine organ where the short-chain fatty acids (SCFAs: acetic acid, lactic acid etc.) and other compounds produced, act like hormones directing the functionality of multiple systems.

Fungi, yeasts, and molds are found mostly on dead or decomposing matter. They have been consumed as food, such as mushrooms, and are used in a variety of food production methods, such as cheese, wine, and beer making. *Acetobacter* are one form of bacteria that ferment the sugars in grapes to produce acetic acid which is also necessary in humans to maintain pH, and for the metabolism of more complex fats and carbohydrates. When fungi, yeast, and mold take up residence in

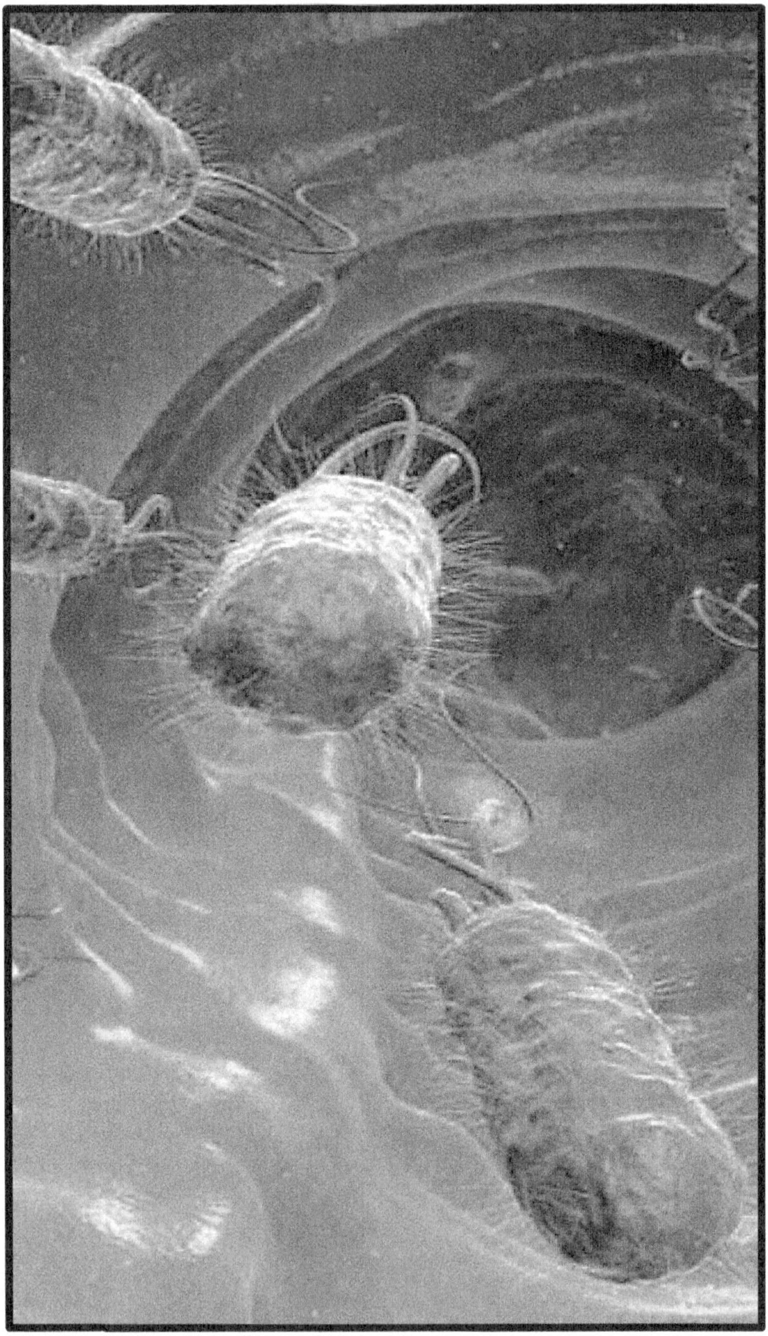

the human system however, they are reflective of a digestive system that is fermenting. These propagate in a highly acidic system (~pH of 5). Rather than facilitating digestion and producing energy in the form of adenosine triphosphate (ATP) through the oxidation of glucose to pyruvic acid in the aerobic respiration of the Krebs cycle, pyruvic acid is fermented by yeast to form lactic acid. *Lactobacillus* are needed to convert lactic acid back to acetic acid to prevent lactic acidosis. When the tight junctions of the intestinal lining are open, these same fungus and molds enter into the body's circulatory system.

Intestinal bacteria are responsive to their environment, the foods that are eaten, systemic pH balance, and oxygen levels. They are also responsive to the stress levels and mental/emotional context of the individual. These bacteria survive within a normal range that fluctuates in relation to daily influences.

> **When the individual and their biome is in balance, health is maintained, systems are properly regulated, cognitive processes are in sync with reality, and vitality is felt.**

When any one of the conditions maintaining balance is disrupted, e.g. prolonged stress, antibiotics, errors in dietary consumption, and toxic exposures such as medication, heavy metals, glyphosate, etc., the biome is correspondingly altered.

Individual bacteria mutate to accommodate to the now hostile environment or populations of new, potentially pathogenic, yet better adapted, species propagate. All this leads to a resultant shift in metabolic by-products, neurotransmitter production, and immune system regulation as these new bacteria become the new operators in the system.

Soil Biome and Agriculture: The health, vitality, and nutritional content of all agricultural crops is dependent upon the health of the soil. Healthy soil is rich in organic matter, fungus, and bacteria and it is teaming with other living organisms that all work in symbiotic relationship to the plants growing in that soil. Seeds germinate under the influence of the soil micro-bacteria and these healthy soil organisms work with the plants growing to facilitate assimilation of the minerals and nutrients from the soil.

Sustainable agricultural practices insist on crop rotation, rest years, and natural weed control and fertilization from livestock to maintain soil health, to have disease resistant crops and give consistently high yields.

Modern agricultural practices have lost these farming techniques opting for mono crops and the reliance upon artificial fertilizers to force growth, and herbicides and pesticides to control 'invasive species' and disease. The result of which has led to tracks of land devoid of a naturally diverse biome, depletion of vital nutrients, changed populations of natural wildlife, and production of food so nutritionally deficient that it needs to be artificially fortified with indigestible synthetic vitamins, in order to satisfy national nutritional guidelines.

Biome in Fetal Development: In humans, the intestinal microbiota has the largest number of bacteria and the greatest number of species, as compared to other areas of the body. The intestinal lining of infants is established in utero by the infant swallowing and excreting the amniotic fluid. In early pregnancy, amniotic fluid is mainly water with electrolytes, but by about the 12-14th week the liquid also contains proteins, carbohydrates, lipids, phospholipids, and urine from the fetus, all of which aid in fetal growth and prepares its intestinal lining to house the necessary commensal bacteria. This amniotic fluid is akin to the primordial sea of abiogenesis and provides the necessary trace minerals and metals that are needed through all stages of not only nutritional and functional fetal development but also those aspects of our soul and being that connects us to the universe within which our consciousness exists.

Assuming the mother has a healthy biome, passage through the birth canal, and the swallowing of the amniotic fluid, mother's bodily fluids, blood, urine, stool, and commensal bacteria introduces the healthy bacterial population vital to the life of the infant and their innate and adaptive immunity. *Lactobacillus*, the predominant bacteria, and the lactic acid produced by them are essential to keep the vagina acidic and free of pathogenic bacteria and yeasts. Suckling at the breast, with contact to the mother's skin and ingesting first colostrum (containing antibodies) and subsequent mother's milk, grounds the transition of the fetus into the outer world. Although breast-fed infants do not show appreciable numbers of bacteria in their stool until after they are weaned, *Bacteroides* and *Lactobacillus* are a part of normal, healthy mother's placental and vaginal microbiome. For the infant, in the first one to two years after birth, this population stabilizes its relationship to the intestinal epithelium and the mucosal barrier secreted by the epithelial cells. The biome and intestinal lining co-develop in a way that renders the intestines tolerant to, and even supportive of, that same biome. Likewise, zonulin (haptoglobin), a protein whose relative concentrations are regulated by the DNA in intestinal immune cells, serves to maintain the tight junctions in this same intestinal lining. By doing so, this lining provides a barrier to pathogenic organisms and compels metabolites to enter the body through the portal vein, the normal route of entry. More importantly this process of discernment on behalf of the intestinal lining correlates relatively to the intellect's ability to discern what is good for you or not. Interestingly, oral exposure to live polio virus in the first weeks of life facilitates this critical regulation of zonulin, preventing a host of potential infections and auto-immune inflammatory responses, thus, preventing an overwhelm on the spleen's ability to clean the plasma.

Gut microorganisms benefit the host by fermenting dietary fiber into short-chain fatty acids (SCFAs), such as acetic acid and butyric acid, which are then absorbed through the intestinal lining for other functions. Intestinal bacteria also play a role in synthesizing the B vitamins and vitamin K, as well as metabolizing bile acids, sterols, and xenobiotics (against life: drugs, pesticides, carcinogens). The gut flora itself appears to also function like an endocrine organ where the short chain fatty acids (SCFAs), and other compounds produced, act like hormones directing the functionality of multiple systems. Tryptophan, the precursor to many neurotransmitters is produced by this same biome.

Evolution of Bacteria: In order to survive fluctuations in environments, bacteria adapt by exchanging genetic material and exchange genes by one of three specialized means: conjugation, transformation, or transduction.[xcv] Bacteria are programed to survive, and they will adapt to do so. They don't really care what they become. Their survival is what is important. Bits of DNA or RNA are like thoughts, one bacterium can exchange thoughts with another bacterium. Bacteria can adapt to live in radioactive soils, oil spills, and under the toxic exposure of glyphosate. While survival of the human animal is dependent upon a bacterial population, how it thrives is dependent on the kind of biome it houses.

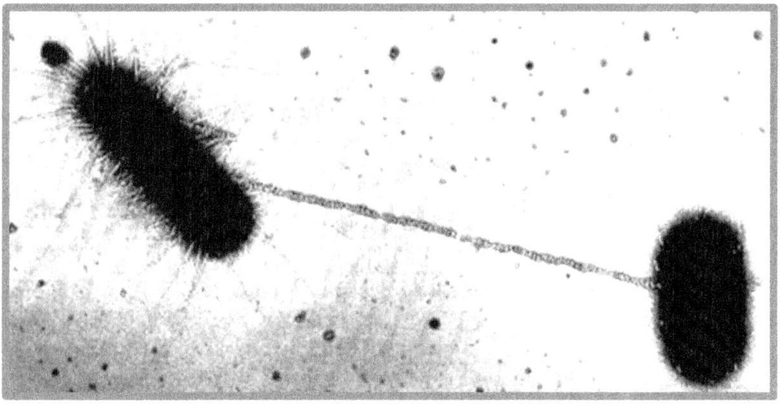

A. Conjugation: the process of exchanging genetic material through cell-to-cell contact (conjugation bridge). The bacteria attach using special hair like structures called pili, and important DNA passes from one cell to another (depicted above). Uptake of this new DNA allows the recipient to adapt to the new environment and provides variations and diversity of the generations of bacteria to follow. This increases the chances that the bacteria will survive environmental changes. Humans, like bacteria, also learn and evolve by sharing bits of information, thoughts, viruses, and DNA.

B. Transformation: the process by which bacteria cells pick up and incorporate DNA from dead bacteria cells of the same or a closely related species. The new DNA enables them to be more adaptive.

C. Transduction: using a virus (small strand of coding DNA) to transfer DNA from one bacterium to another. Viruses called bacteriophages can be added into the bacterial hosts DNA. This is one way to get bacteria to make large amounts of proteins for research and medicine, e.g. to produce human insulin or other hormones, or how bacteria learn to clean up oil spills.

Viruses, Viral Mutation, and the Intestinal Biome: By design, RNA viruses have developed alongside humanity's evolution as a way to modulate and facilitate not only metabolic functions, but also to active immunological responses that intern activate developmental and societal transformations. RNA viruses are also able to mutate based on the self-regulating feedback loops opting for one genetic expression over another. The selection process is what has enabled the science of artificial genetic modification.

These replication methods are important to consider for bacteria and viruses when the hosts' intestinal environment becomes too toxic and the healthy bacteria become pathological only in order to survive. Accordingly, infectious disease agents are intended to activate the built-in survival mechanism of the human host by way of a fever, localization, and discharge. When, and only when, the immune system cycles completely through these stages immunity is generated and the beneficial process that infectious agent was intended to impart can be actualized.

Normally the human animal host utilizes its immune system to keep potentially pathogenic bacterial populations in check. A fever and subsequent discharge are necessary to bring about the detoxification process needed to allow a healthy biome to reestablish itself. Suppression of fevers cripples the self-correcting duty of the immune system.

Glyphosate Toxicity and the Biome: Because glyphosate disrupts the shikimate-acid pathway in all *Bifidobacteria* in the intestinal biome, all who consume glyphosate contaminated foods will be affected. There is no escape. Disruption in the gut biome of gestating mothers and infants has more detrimental outcomes as the development of a healthy gut lining in utero and early infancy determines the subsequent health of all systems as that child develops. Because glyphosate suppresses the immune system through interference with the adenosine receptor sites, the activity of RNA viruses induces a host of immunological consequences.

Glyphosate Effects in the Biome:[xcvi]

i. Glyphosate induces selective bactericide preference to lacto-fermenting bacteria by interfering with their shikimate-acid pathway.
ii. The shikimate-acid pathway of all lacto-fermenting bacteria is disturbed due to interference in the creation of EPSP synthase. This enzyme is essential for the creation of Cytochrome P450-Enzymes (heme-dependent enzymes)needed in the liver to chelate heavy metals, create bile acids and bile salts for fat emulsification, and in tryptophan production.
iii. Lacto-fermenting bacteria are also responsible for the synthesis of methionine, the precursor to glutathione an important antioxidant.
iv. Displacement of normal bacterial populations leads to overgrowth of pathogenic bacteria or *Candida.* More specifically *Bifidobacteria* are displaced resulting in overgrowth of *Clostridium difficile*, non-beneficial *E. coli* species, *Salmonella*, *Pseudomonas*, or *Candida* species. These species have the capacity to mutate and further develop antibiotic and glyphosate resistance by substituting their need for glycine by interjecting alanine, thereby rendering them glyphosate resistant. *E. coli* and *salmonella* can pump out glyphosate from within their cells. Methicillin resistant *staphylococcus* (MRSA) is equally resistant to glyphosate.
v. *Acetobacter* can metabolize glyphosate. Glyphosate toxicity invites over-population of this family of bacteria that synthesizes acetic acid which would be necessary in a high lactic acid environment when *Bifidobacteria* populations are reduced.
vi. *Bifidobacteria* are preferentially killed by glyphosate. These bacteria are responsible for the conversion of bile acids to bile salts and the creation of methionine.
vii. Yeast/*Candida* overgrowth, however, can help in the detoxification process of heavy metals that the cells can no longer affect due to nutritional and enzyme dysfunction and lack of

creation of glutathione. High *Candida* environments produce alcohol through their formation process.

viii. Glyphosate encourages the growth of the bacteria *Desulfovibrio* which are normal soil bacteria and are often used in bioremediation due to their ability to transform toxins. However, in the body they transform mercury in to methylmercury which increases its toxicity.

ix. *Clostridia*, *Bacteriodetes*, and *Desulfovibrio* species, during lactic acid fermentation, produce a high amount of propionic acid (PPA) and its related short-chain fatty acids (SCFAs). Elevated propionic acid levels can induce widespread effects on gut, brain, and behavior. Excess PPA and related SCFAs induces abnormal motor movements, repetitive interests, electrographic changes, cognitive deficits, perseveration, and impaired social interactions. Propionic acid induces neurochemical changes, including innate neuroinflammation, increased oxidative stress, glutathione depletion, and altered phospholipid/acylcarnitine profiles. PPA has bioactive effects on neurotransmitter systems, intracellular acidification/calcium release, fatty acid metabolism, tight junction gating, immune function, and alteration of gene expression.[xcvii]

x. Normal stomach pH is around 6. Small intestinal pH increases to about 7.4 and then reduces again in the lower intestine to 5.7 and finally increases to 6.7 in the rectum. Glyphosate's impact on the lacto-fermenting bacteria results in reduced levels of acetic acid which is a short-chain fatty acid produced by those bacteria from the oxidation of lactic acid. Acetic acid helps to maintain an alkaline pH and serves in the digestion of fats and carbohydrates. Glyphosate encourages an acidic environment (low pH) thereby encouraging *Candida* overgrowth. A healthy *Bifidobacteria* population in the small intestine keeps it in a more alkaline state (pH: 7-7.4).

xi. Acetate, acetic acid combined with an earth metal, is necessary to control overgrowth of yeasts and molds. Lactic acid is oxidized to acetic acid, then estered to form acetate. *Lactobacillus* or *Bifidobacteria* convert lactic acid to acetic acid thus controlling yeast and mold populations.

xii. Reduced *lactobacillus* encourages *Clostridium difficile* over-growth. The toxins released by the *Clostridia* species causes increase in pain levels and cerebral inflammation through depletion of the enzyme tyrosine hydroxylase. A deficiency of tyrosine hydroxylase leads to impaired conversion of dopamine to epinephrine of and norepinephrine. Excess dopamine manifests as progressive encephalopathy and a poor prognosis and neuronal burnout. Increased glutamate level is also a result of depleted tyrosine hydroxylase. As a result, the individual is in a constant state of excitement, cerebral inflammation, pain, and distress. This can also lead to schizophrenia.

xiii. Folate (B9) is a product of the shikimate-acid pathway from *Bifidobacteria* in the intestinal biome, or the food we eat and is an essential ingredient for neurodevelopment and neurotransmitter creation. The brain needs folate (B9), not folic acid which is the synthetic form. Glyphosate kills the bacteria that produce folate (B9). Synthetic folic acid is difficult to methylate. The enzyme methylenetetrahydrofolate reductase (MTHFR) needed for the vitamin C dependent folic acid to folate (B9) conversion pathway is also glycine dependent. In those with MTHFR gene mutations this enzyme is not made. Excess folic acid is toxic to the liver and blood stream. Those individuals with the MTHFR gene mutations, whereby they cannot convert folic acid to folate (B9) or even methylate folate (B9) need to consume foods with high amounts of folate (B9) in addition to methionine supplementation to have the building blocks necessary to create sufficient neurotransmitters for healthy neurodevelopment. As glyphosate disrupts the shikimate-acid pathway in *Bifidobacteria* a natural consequence of glyphosate toxicity is folate (B9) deficiency.

xiv. Deficiency in folate (B9) and cobalamin (B12) leads to hyperhomocysteinemia due to the need of B9 and B12 to convert homocysteine to cystine in the methionine methylation pathway. Increased homocysteine levels increase the risk of cardiovascular disease, Alzheimer's, dementia, declining memory, poor concentration and judgment, and lowered mood. Women with high homocysteine levels find it harder to conceive and are at risk from repeated early miscarriage. Hyperhomocysteinemia has also been linked to migraines, diabetes, and osteoporosis.

xv. Glyphosate causes interference in the glycine dependent digestive enzymes trypsin, pepsin and lipase specifically. The wheat proteins that form gluten, glutenins and gliadins, need trypsin to be digested. Fats need lipase. Hybridized wheat is especially high in gliadins which are relatively undigestible and instigate intestinal inflammation.

xvi. This class of wheat proteins, gliadins, which now cannot be digested, triggers the intestinal lining to upregulate zonulin excretion more so than . This is a signaling molecule which normally critically regulates the tight junctions of the gut. Upregulation of zonulin opens the tight junctions in the intestinal lining and allows for the trafficking of bacteria, viral particles, antigens, and metabolites into the submucosa leading to system-wide inflammatory conditions.[xcviii] The enzyme trypsin is also needed to metabolize zonulin. Natural contraction of live polio in early childhood, an enterovirus, contracted via the fecal oral route, downregulates zonulin signaling and serves to maintain the tight junctions against other infectious agents throughout life.[xcix]

xvii. Disruption in the healthy bacterial-dependent mucosal lining of the intestines leads to inflammation and breakage of the tight junctions between the lining's cells. Inflammatory cytokines as a result of this breakage results in leaky gut syndrome, inflammatory bowel syndrome, and Crohn's disease. Via these gaps in the intestinal lining, undigested food passes directly into the circulatory system bypassing the normal route of portal vein to the liver.

xviii. Undigested gliadin passes into the blood stream through the leaky gut causing system-wide inflammatory responses (Celiac disease). Celiac disease increases the risk of non-Hodgkin's lymphoma.

xix. Bacteria and *Candida* can also pass through these breaks, bypassing the immune system cells in the intestinal lining, resulting in systemic bacterial infections and systemic *Candida*.

xx. Leaky gut results in leaky brain where by these proteins and pathogens now attach to and degrade the blood-brain barrier exciting the inflammatory response in the brains' immune system resulting in cerebral inflammation and neuropsychiatric disorders.

xxi. By adding the inflammatory agents of infectious disease in vaccines along with aluminum adjuvants into infants' immune systems, in addition to inflammation already set up by glyphosate contaminated food, brain inflammation is exacerbated.

xxii. Glyphosate causes interference of the creation of the glycine dependent protein myosin which is coded in the RNA by GGC. Myosin is the smooth muscle protein involved in the contraction and relaxation of the muscles of the large intestine, gallbladder, heart, and uterus. Its action allows for peristalsis of the bowels and in the gallbladder's release of bile acids. Calcium exchange through the calcium channels in muscle cell membranes initiates activation of myosin contraction and relaxation. Myosin has an essential glycine residue which, in high concentrations of glyphosate, gets replaced with the amino acid alanine. If 2% of the glycine in a muscle fiber is replaced by alanine the contractibility goes down by 50%. Inactivity of the bowel, gallbladder, heart, and uterus leads to disfunction of these organs. As glyphosate also leaches calcium, deficiency, and its relationship with myosin, also contributes to intestinal smooth muscle inactivity. Individuals with chronic fatigue syndrome (CFS), most often induced by latent Epstein-Barr virus (EBV), present symptoms related to the relative ratio of myosin fiber types in skeletal muscles (slow or fast twitch muscles). This includes soreness, easy fatigability of the muscles, and increased lactate accumulation in the muscles. Suppression of the immune system by activation of adenosine receptor sites triggers latent EBV and compounds system wide depletion of myosin activity.[c]

xxiii. Insufficient bile release and poor gut motility can lead to small intestinal bacterial overgrowth (SIBO), excess *Bifidobacteria* growing in the wrong portion of the intestines. This leads to the development of food sensitivities and an increase in lactic acid and elevated histamine. This compounds intestinal inflammation and leaky gut syndrome. SIBO is common in children with autism. It is also a complication of Celiac disease or in those individuals who have previously taken a lot of antibiotics.

xxiv. Disruption of the biome reduces the conjugation of bile acids to bile salts in the intestines. Bile salts are needed to emulsify fat.

xxv. Disruption in biome leads to serotonin deficiency because of the disruption of the shikimate-acid pathway and the resultant deficiency of EPSP synthase needed to create tryptophan which is the precursor to serotonin and other neurotransmitters. Additionally, macrophages that come in to engulf the opportunistic bacteria soak up the tryptophan to make kynurenine as an inflammatory agent against these opportunistic bacteria.

xxvi. Deficiencies in serotonin and interference with its receptors sites leads to an increase in pain levels. Serotonin also induces motility of the intestines. Deficiency can also lead to depression, insomnia and constipation.

xxvii. Glyphosate toxicity of the mother and infant and resultant biome disruption and intestinal lining damage set the stage for vaccine introduced infectious disease agents to further propel the inflammatory responses in the brain. By their nature some infectious agents are neurotoxic, as they engage acetylcholine receptors (*Clostridia* species) or produce inflammation, spasms, or paralysis in the central nervous system or gastrointestinal track. (*Clostridium tetani-Tetanus* toxin (zinc dependent receptors), Whooping cough-*Pertussis* toxin, *Diphtheria* toxin, Poliovirus, Measles virus, Chickenpox virus (Herpes), etc.). Vaccination imports these viruses and compounds this problem[ci]

xxviii. Hemagglutinin is a protein found in the measles virus (measles is an RNA Virus). Measles viruses, and associated proteins, incubated on glyphosate mediums, also uptake glyphosate into their structure. The MMR vaccine derived glyphosate contaminated measles protein is difficult to breakdown. The antibodies produced as an immune response from the vaccine antigen target the measles hemagglutinin will also attack the brain's myelin due to its similarity in structure to hemagglutinin. This inflammatory response is further propagated by aluminum adjuvant toxicity and all other glyphosate toxicity issues mentioned beforehand that encourage cerebral inflammation. The addition of mercury and aluminum in vaccines further drives neural toxicity and inflammatory responses.[cii] This molecular mimicry phenomena is exemplified through vaccines that are incubated on aborted fetal tissue cell lines: the similarity of the DNA in these tissues to our own drives auto-immune conditions.

xxix. The conclusion of this trajectory, with the potentiation of contamination of the food supply by glyphosate, the resultant destruction of the intestinal biome, immune system crippling, or auto-immune disease due to the toxic over load of vaccines with RNA viruses, and accompanying aluminum adjuvants and mercury preservatives, in developing immune systems is bleak.[ciii]

Comments: We need bacteria and viruses to be healthy. We are a compilation of bacterial and viral strands of DNA that work in a cohesive fashion without our intervention. The healthy functionality of our innate immune system is needed to keep it all in balance. By design, our DNA has created an immune system that works in relationship to the environment we inhabit and knows how to do all this without us even being conscious.

By the natural order of things, humans and animals have lived on this planet for thousands of years prior to the introduction of genetically modified organisms, glyphosate, or vaccines. We are of this planet and have survived in accordance to the laws of nature.

Pathogens have evolved over time in relationship with humans. They have come and gone in epidemics and scourges based on varying collective susceptibilities in those human populations. These pathogens have shaped cultures, religious behaviors, and rituals throughout history.

Pathogens have acted as checks and balances in the human population based upon human frailties and errors of thought or living. The action of pathogens are pressure release valves for situations and environments not conducive to sustaining human life, either for the individual, or the larger population. These disease inducing agents also can serve as teachers by activating adaptive responses that encourage survivability. Those with poor nutrition, living in over-crowded or unsanitary conditions, or those under certain political and social pressures have a much greater susceptibility to contracting disease.

The immune response generated is deigned to draw out the survivability of that being. The weaker, the old, and the young, are at greater risk of complications in these disease processes. Collectively this natural evolution process serves to maintain individuals and populations in health.

While it is not the pathogen itself that directly causes complications, it is the reaction, or lack of reaction, of the human body to the pathogen that dictates the course the disease will follow. Healthy immunological responses drive greater adaptability of the individual

We can't live in a glass bubble removed from bacteria and viruses as we have evolved from this compilation that governs the entire operating system of our body. These same bacteria and viruses are a part of the living breathing biome of Gaia, the living breathing earth. If we try to remove these bacterial or viral agents from our existence, we do not exist. If we pollute the planet and kill off the bacteria symbiotic to proper nutrition in plants, or cripple our immune systems with vaccines and antibiotics, and consume glyphosate corrupted food which destroys all healthy bacteria and our intestinal barrier, the only outcome

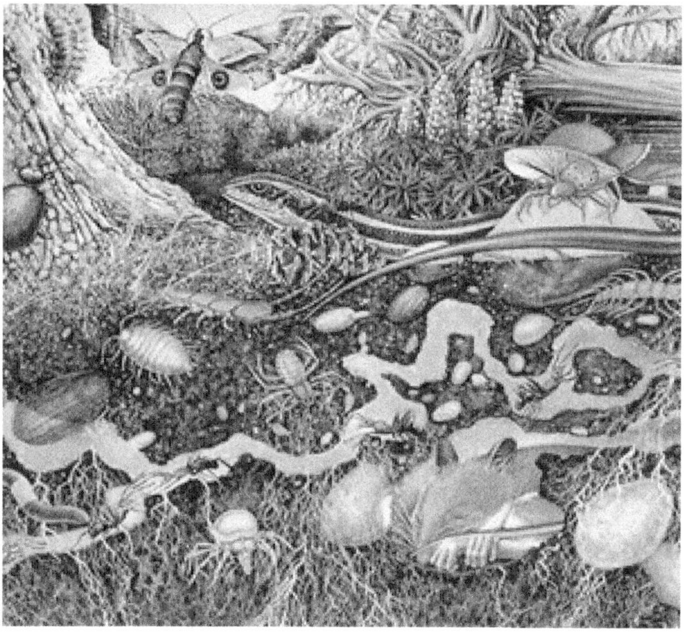

is an under-nourished and over-inflamed body, riddled with pathological bacteria and activated retroviral strands that become disease producing operators.

Accordingly, our immune system is a survival mechanism for our bodies and rectifies our vital force energy and our ego (limited self-perception) with the forces of reality or hereditary. When our ego is out of sync with these forces (unable or unwilling to see nature as it is), disease producing bacteria and viruses come along to activate the survival mechanism necessary to propel us towards life.

Conversely, if left to its own devices, the earth upon which we live, obedient to nature's laws, will heal itself from the wounds we have inflicted upon her. The soil too, as a living breathing organism that contributes to the oxygen we breath, can also work to clean up toxins, radiation, heavy metals, pollution and the damages from acid rain. Better adapted microbia will take up this work.

Survival is not only an immunological process but also cognitive. The cognitive aspect is to look within and see what facets of how we live, and who we think we are, work against our true nature. It is this wounded-ego-based thinking that is behind polluting the environment - if we loved ourselves, we would not poison ourselves. How we perceive and treat the external environment is a mirror of how we perceive and treat ourselves. The potential disease entities that we may contract serve to activate our immune system towards the truth of our susceptibilities and psychological/ physiological encumbrances in order for us to survive.

The tight junctions of the intestinal lining are the operators of discernment; that process by which we determine what is good for our body and that which is not. Discernment is both physiological and psychological. It is the ability to stand up in ones' own power in the face of fear. Normally if we ingest food that is bad for us, we will eject that food through vomiting or diarrhea. Normally before putting food in our mouth we first look, smell, and taste to see if it would be good for us or not. The resultant system-wide reflexive action stimulated in our body would either induce desire or aversion for that food. Failure to discriminate and discern what we put in our body leads to multiple levels of suffering and the likelihood of being controlled, dominated, overwhelmed and subjugated to the power of others and the foods we eat. Somehow, glyphosate, and the food manufacturing industry has modified our ability to appropriately discern what is good for us or not. Not only with regards to what we put in our body, but also with regards to commercial news, misguided thinking, or manipulation of science to justify the use of glyphosate and genetically modified food products.

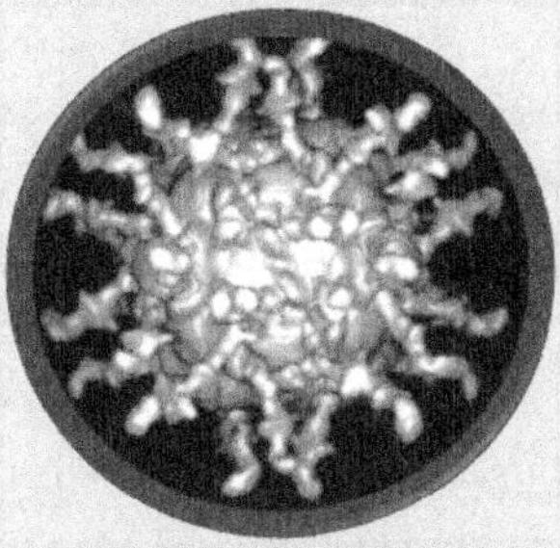

Polio virus: an RNA enterovirus intended to be contracted in infancy to down regulate the tight junctions of the intestinal lining while it is maturing.

If we are willing to put toxins in our body what would stop us from doing the same to the earth? It we are uncomfortable inside our own skin, the results of the DNA that coded our creation, or repulsed by the intestinal bacteria we need to facilitate our digestive processes, what would stop us from trying to destroying ourselves, all bacteria, and the desire to tinker with or contaminate our DNA?

Polio, measles, and chickenpox are viruses that are meant to be contracted in childhood to activate that survival prerogative and rectify the strength of our vital force with that of the environment.[civ, cv, cvi] While each of these diseases pose specific risks, the immune systems of healthy children who move through the respective disease processes activated have increased vitality.[cvii] Vaccines that block access to wild-virus-infective processes do nothing for the survival dictates of the immune system. Homeoprophylaxis, the introduction of the potentized preparation of disease agents, offers the opportunity to be exposed to the energetics of the disease and to capitulate the associated adaptive immunological response that stimulates immunity.

Another example of this is PANDAS (Pediatric Auto-immune Neuropsychiatric Disorders Associated with *Streptococcal* infections). This is driven by the use of antibiotics to kill *Streptococcal* bacteria. In their place, *Clostridium difficile* or *Candida* overgrowth occurs. Over time as the normal bacterial balance attempts to reestablish itself (including healthy *streptococcal* bacteria) a fever develops. This fever is asking the individual to get their internal environment in order so as to live in harmony with *Bifidobacteria* populations (*Streptococcus* is a lacto-fermenting bacteria).

I am happy my immune system knows how to get a fever and recover. We all need that. I am happy to know that my mental and emotional experience is a direct extension of the inner workings of my immune system in relation to my biome and the discerning ability of my intestinal lining. If one's immune system is so broken that you cannot do that, what does that say about your ability to survive not only physically, but psychologically?

Vaccines and glyphosate have created a whole generation of children unable to reconcile the co-infections of multiple vaccine introduced viral and bacterial agents. They are suffering from ADD, ADHD, autism, and pervasive developmental delays and will be dependent on the social service system their entire life because glyphosate has taken

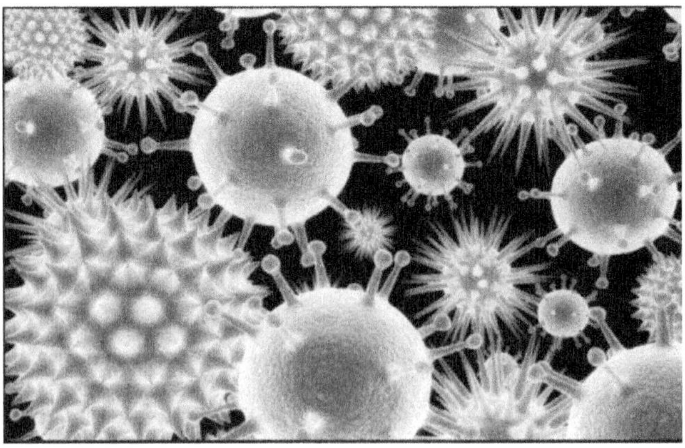

over their entire operating system. They are nutrient starved, their DNA has been dysregulated, their biomes and intestinal linings are destroyed, hormonal and neurotransmitter levels are out of balance, and the survival mechanism of their immune system has been disabled.[cviii] If you put those kids out in the street, desert, forest, or on a mountain top they will die. Not from infectious disease, but because they do not know how to cognitively think, discern, or survive in the natural environment.

---

xcv Bio Teacher. Bacteria. LC Biology Class 1, Organism. http://leavingbio.net/bacteria/.

xcvi Seneff, Stephanie. Glyphosate+ Aluminum+ Mercury + Glutamate= Autism. AutismOne Media. June 1, 2018. https://www.youtube.com/watch?v=OL9mr599hb0.

xcvii Derrick F. MacFabe, MD. Short-chain fatty acid fermentation products of the gut microbiome: implications in autism spectrum disorders. Microbobial Ecolology in Health and Disease. 2012. 10.3402/mehd.v23i0.19260. https://www.ncbi.nlm.nih.gov/pmc/articles/PMC3747729/.

xcviii Visser, Jeroen; Rozing, Jan; Sapone, Anna; Lammers, Karen; Fasano, Alessio (2009-05-01). Tight Junctions, Intestinal Permeability, and Autoimmunity Celiac Disease and Type 1 Diabetes Paradigms. Annals of the New York Academy of Sciences. 1165: 195–205.

xcix Christine Stabell Benn. How vaccines train the immune system in ways no one expected. TEDxAarhus. https://www.youtube.com/watch?v=_d8PNlXHJ48.

c Pietrangelo T, Toniolo L, Paoli A, Fulle S, Puglielli C, Fanò G, Reggiani C. Functional characterization of muscle fibres from patients with chronic fatigue syndrome: case-control study. Int. J. Immunopatholy Pharmacoly. 2009 Apr-Jun;22(2):427-36. https://www.ncbi.nlm.nih.gov/pubmed/19505395.

cii Derrick F. MacFabe, MD. Short-chain fatty acid fermentation products of the gut microbiome: implications in autism spectrum disorders. Microbobial Ecolology in Health and Disease. 2012. 10.3402/mehd.v23i0.19260. https://www.ncbi.nlm.nih.gov/pmc/articles/PMC3747729/.

ciii Dr. Nancy Swanson. The Autism Epidemic: Data show correlations between increase in neurological diseases and GMOs. 4/6/2013. http://myfoodstuff.net/application/files/1514/9046/2512/GMO-6_neurological_disease.pdf.

civ Birch, Kate. The Story of Measles. July 30, 2018 https://freeandhealthychildren.org/2018/07/30/the-story-of-measles-2/.

cv Birch, Kate. Chickenpox Ensures Survival. Aug 1. 2018. https://freeandhealthychildren.org/2018/08/01/chickenpox-ensures-survival/.

cvi Christine Stabell Benn. How vaccines train the immune system in ways no one expected. TEDxAarhus. https://www.youtube.com/watch?v=_d8PNlXHJ48.

cvii Ibid.

cviii Stephine Libran, Juliette Igier. Genetically Modified Children. Cinema Libre Studio. 2017. https://store.cinemalibrestore.com/genetically-modified-children-dvd.html. https://vimeo.com/285569497.

7. Glyphosate, Neurotransmitters, and Hormones

Neurotransmitters and Hormones: Both play a critical and vital role in shaping everyday human experience and multiple organ system functions in the body. They are endogenous protein messengers, (made from within the body) that enable the transmission of signals between receptor sites on various cell types.

Types of transmissions include one neuron (nerve cell) or glandular cell to another's target receptor site on the membrane of a neuron, a muscle cell, immune cell, or other glandular cell. Once engaged in the receptor site of the receiving cell the neurotransmitter or hormone directs (suppresses or excites) the action or functions in that cell. All these actions and reactions take place through activation of the G-protein coupled receptor (GPCR) sites, glycine/calcium dependent channels or cholinergic receptors in the cell membranes of target cells in or outside the brain.

Neurotransmitters: In the brain neurotransmitters are released from synaptic vesicles in one neuron during a synapses into the synaptic cleft, where they are received by neurotransmitter receptors on the target neurons. In health, many neurotransmitters are synthesized from simple and plentiful precursors such as amino acids, which are readily available from a healthy diet and healthy biome. In health, they only require a small number of biosynthetic steps for conversion. Their exact numbers are unknown, but more than 200 chemical messengers have been uniquely identified.

Tryptophan is an essential aromatic amino acid that must be synthesized in the bacteria that we host. Tryptophan is a precursor for the creation of the monoamine neurotransmitters: serotonin (wellbeing and happiness), melatonin (sleep inducer): and niacin (B3) (precursor of coenzymes necessary for the catabolism of fats, carbohydrates, proteins and alcohol; it is also necessary for fatty acid and cholesterol synthesis as well as cell signaling and DNA repair).

Tryptophan is a precursor to phenylalanine, another essential aromatic amino acid, which is a precursor for the tyrosine. Tryptophan and phenylalanine production is contingent on the glycine-dependent enzyme EPSP synthase needed for their coding. EPSP synthase is created by the lacto-fermenting bacteria living in our intestines. If glyphosate does not kill the bacteria outright it will supplant the glycine in the coding for EPSP synthase making it inoperable. Both results of which will lead to a deficiency in the tryptophan and phenylalanine that all neurotransmitters are dependent upon.

Tyrosine is created from phenylalanine by hydroxylation with the enzyme phenylalanine hydroxylase. Tyrosine is also ingested directly from dietary protein. Catecholamines are neurotransmitters derived from tyrosine. Catecholamine-secreting cells use several reactions to convert tyrosine serially to L-DOPA and then to dopamine (pleasure response). Depending on the cell type, dopamine may be further converted to norepinephrine or even further converted to epinephrine. Catecholamines can serve as neurotransmitters, transferring signals from neuron to neuron, as well as hormones, which regulate physiological functions in specific organs such as your heartbeat and breathing rate.

Within the biological process of neurotransmitter balance is the living breathing human being, capable of sensing, perceiving, comprehending and rational understanding of the world he inhabits.

Hormones: These are endogenous protein messengers which are secreted from the glands of the endocrine system that, based on built in regulating feedback loops. These maintain and control the functioning of the glandular system, their target organs, and functions.

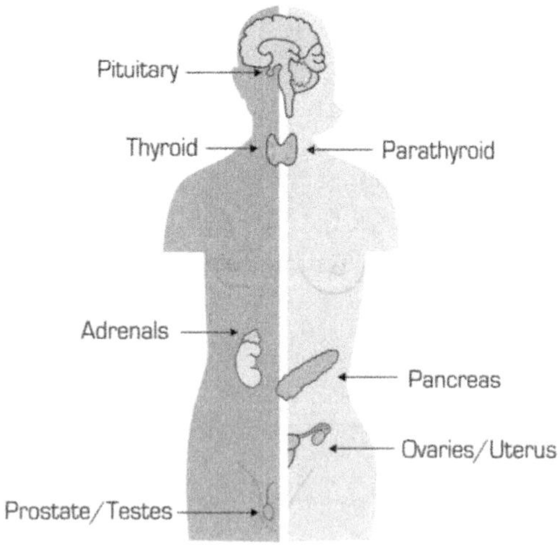

The hypothalamic-pituitary-adrenal axis which governs fight or flight, and hypothalamic-pituitary-thyroid axis, which governs metabolism and growth, are functional neurotransmitter/hormonal excretory and receptor site systems. Nerve impulses directed along the vagus nerve, coordinate communication between the glands in the nervous, gastrointestinal, and endocrine systems, the hormones secreted, and the organs that respond to those secretions. Hormones secreted include epinephrine, adrenaline, androgens (estrogen, testosterone, etc.), thyroid stimulating hormone (TSH), triiodothyronine (T3), thyroxine (T4), zonulin, and others.

The Vagus Nerve: Governing three main functions which all connect to the communication systems involved with caretaking:

1. To slow down the heart rate.
2. To calm the effects of any fight or flight autonomic nervous system activity, the body's response to any kind of stress.
3. To initiate the release of oxytocin, a neuropeptide and hormone, that plays a role in love, trust, intimacy, and devotion. Oxytocin is made in the hypothalamus and released by the posterior pituitary.

The vagus nerve gets activated whenever we engage in our higher emotions: altruism, kindness, and compassion. Activation of the vagus nerve helps to nurture universal love in a person and a greater acceptance of differences between the self and the other. If oxytocin is the 'love hormone,' as it is generally referred to, the vagus nerve is the 'love nerve.' When activated, when we show compassion or gratitude, it's also the healing nerve. Oxytocin in combination with choline and inositol facilities the cascade of physiological reactions that induce orgasm.

Pancreatic excretion and the control of glucagon, thyroxine, and androgen levels are critically regulated by the GPCR sites in the hypothalamus. If the critical balance of all hormones is maintained, life occurs unassisted by any medical intervention. Critically regulated, the neurotransmitters and hormones necessary for fetal and childhood development, sexual function, growth and metabolism, and healthy mental and emotional experience in life, operate within normal ranges.

Sympathetic nervous system influence in the body

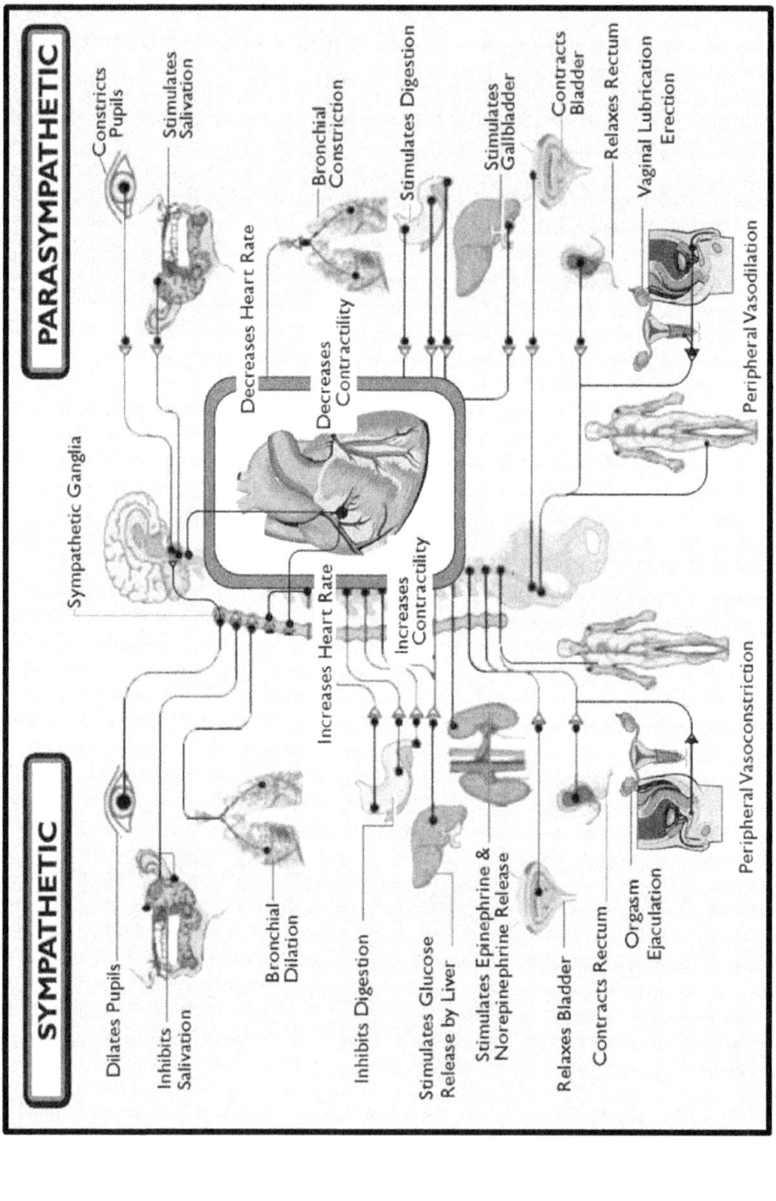

Norepinephrine: functions as a hormone and transmitter. It works to mobilize the brain and body for action in fight or flight responses of the sympathetic nervous system. In the brain, norepinephrine increases arousal and alertness, promotes vigilance, enhances formation and retrieval of memory, and focuses attention. It also increases restlessness and anxiety. In the rest of the body, norepinephrine acts hormonally to increase heart rate and blood pressure. In the fight or flight response it triggers the release of glucose from energy stores, increases blood flow to skeletal muscle, and reduces blood flow to the gastrointestinal lining.

Norepinephrine acts by binding to and activating noradrenergic GPCR receptors located on the cell surface of the adrenal medulla. This stimulates the adrenal cortex to release epinephrine (adrenaline). These systems work in coordination with each other to maintain balance within the individual in relationship to the stresses and environment that they live in.

Glutamate and GABA: L-glutamine is a conditionally essential amino acid sourced from food and synthesized in the body. It is the precursor for the production of the neurotransmitters Glutamate (excitatory) and GABA (inhibitory action in the mature brain-memory and learning, excitatory in the developing brain). The balance of these two neurotransmitters is critical for optimal brain function.

Glutamate cannot cross the blood-brain barrier unassisted, but it is actively transported into the nervous system by a high affinity transport system controlled by the glycine dependent calcium channels in the blood-brain barrier. This transport system maintains calcium concentrations in the intercranial fluids at constant levels. The balance between neural excitation and neural inhibition is crucial to healthy cognition and behavior.

Excess glutamate leads to neurotoxicity in the brain resulting in hyperactivity, cerebral inflammation, possible seizures, or schizophrenia. In the immune system however, glutamate also helps boost T cell activity by activating the glutamate GPCR sites on Immune cells, stimulating antibodies to neutralize viruses and pathological bacteria. Conversely, retroviruses and immunological stimulation from vaccine aluminum adjuvants can compound glutamate driven cerebral inflammation. L-glutamine helps to tame inflammatory cytokines. Conversion to L-glutamine with glutamine synthetase (GS) serves to detox the brain of glutamate by transporting excess ammonia to the liver to be converted into other amino acids, nucleotides, sugars and urea.

Inside the brain glutamate and GABA levels are maintained by an efficient concentration feedback loop controlling their respective balance. The functionality of glutamate receptor channels relies upon sodium while GABA receptors rely upon chlorine.

Acetylcholine (ACh): A cholinergic signaling agent in the autonomic nervous system. It is an ester of acetic acid and choline. It acts at the neuromuscular junctions of motor neurons to activate muscles (spasm, contraction, and relaxation) and as a neuromodulator playing an important role in arousal, attention, memory and motivation. It acts as a neurotransmitter and neuromodulator and is synthesized in the brain from choline and acetyl coenzyme A. Acetic acid is derived from the fermentation of sugars by *Acetobacter*. Choline is an essential nutrient that must be derived from the food we eat and is also implicit in the transsulphuration methylation pathway.

Choline along with cobalamin (B12) and folate (B9) is essential to the neurulation process. ACh and the enzymes choline acetyltransferase (ChAT) (needed in its synthesis) and acetylcholinesterase (AChE) (for its degradation), have been traced back to early origins of unicellular bacteria and eukaryotes. ACh effects a range of symptoms from paralysis to convulsions, salivation and perspiration, to endocrine function depending on which GPCR sites are activated.

The vagus nerve is the super highway for cholinergic signaling activity. Nicotinic acetylcholine receptors (nAChRs), particularly responsive to nicotine, are Na^+, K^+, and Ca_2^+ ion channels that conduct nerve impulses from the brain to muscles targeting contractibility. Muscarinic acetylcholine receptors (mAChRs) are classified as M1 through M6 receptor sites. These sites are responsible for the regulation of a number of functions including endocrine and exocrine secretions from cells and mucous membranes (perspiration, salivation, lubrication, emesis (vomiting) and diarrhea), heart contraction and rate, vasodilation, bronchospasm, pupil accommodation and smooth muscle contraction and coordination. Agonists to mAChR sites are ACh, muscarine (*Amanita muscacria* mushroom alkaloid), pilocarpine (alkaloid from the *Pilocarpus* plant genus; *Rutaceae* family (scented Rue, or Citrus plants) and physostigmine (from the *Leguminosae* family (soybeans, peas, lentils, chickpeas).

This means that these alkaloids have the ability to induce paralysis, increased salivation, convulsions, and such. Atropine, hyoscyamine scopolamine (plant alkaloids) and mamba toxins (snake venom from the *Mamba* genus) are antagonists meaning that these alkaloids and toxins breakdown ACh, releasing the receptor sites and arresting the condition.

ACh is also a neurotransmitter in the autonomic nervous system, that acts both as an internal transmitter for the sympathetic nervous system and as the final product released in the parasympathetic nervous system (affecting rest and metabolism). It is an antagonist to adrenaline in its

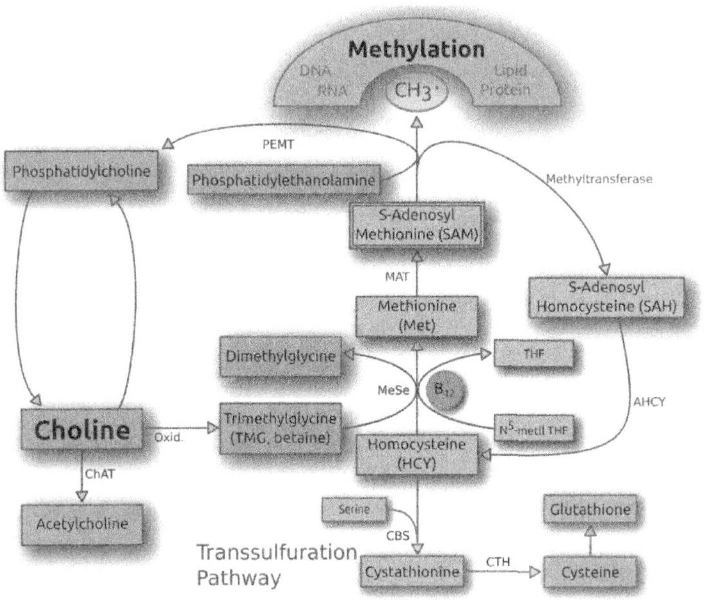

relation to the parasympathetic nervous system. The brain contains several cholinergic stimulated areas, each with distinct functions; playing important roles in arousal, sleep, attention, memory and motivation.

Histamine as a Neurotransmitter: Histamine is involved in local immune responses, as well as regulating physiological function in the gut. It also acts as a neurotransmitter for the brain and spinal cord regulating sleep-wake cycles, appetite, memory, and stress response.

Glyphosate Interferes with:

i. Glyphosate acts as a disruptor of calcium channel receptors. Calcium deficiencies interferes with the functionality of the calcium channels of presynaptic neurons limiting the release of the neurotransmitter signaling proteins glutamate, GABA, ACh, dopamine, and norepinephrine.
ii. Glutamate is metabolized to L-glutamine and ammonia by glutamine synthetase (GS), preferentially activated by magnesium (Mg). Manganese, cobalt and iron will also active this enzyme based on pH values and relative concentrations of the ions. Glyphosate causes deficiency in any one of these minerals limiting the metabolism of glutamate. Increased glutamate leads to hyperactivity, promotes cerebral excitation, and autistic expression.
iii. Glyphosate driven tryptophan deficiency leads to serotonin deficiency and dysregulation of the serotonin GPCR sites which deleteriously effects wellbeing and happiness resulting in an increase in pain/lowering of the pain threshold and increased constipation. Problems with the serotonin pathway are linked to obsessive compulsive disorders (OCD), anxiety disorders, and depression.[cix]
iv. Glyphosate induced depletion of the enzyme tyrosine hydroxylase needed for the breakdown of dopamine, the pleasure and reward response neurotransmitter, leads to neuronal burnout, increased pain, and progressive encephalopathy. Excess dopamine is connected to hallucinations and schizophrenia, defects in memory, motivation, emotion, reward, desire, and addictive behaviors.

Furthermore, increased glutamate levels in combination with excess dopamine compounds the risk of schizophrenia.[cx]

v. Deficiencies of dopamine from a phenylalanine deficiency (from lack of *Bifidobacteria-* and *Lactobacillus*), leads to neuron death, and dysregulation of the hypothalamus-pituitary pathway effecting hormonal control of pregnancy and nurturing instincts.[cxi]

vi. Deficiencies in dopamine also leads to insufficient epinephrine and adrenaline production, adrenal burnout, and dysregulation of the hypothalamic-pituitary-adrenal/-thyroid axes.[cxii]

vii. ACh works with histamine to contract muscles in the lungs. Glyphosate toxicity suppresses AChE transcription which is important for acetyl cholinergic signaling inhibition by degrading excess ACh. AChE is an enzyme in the carboxylesterase family of enzymes which are the primary target of organophosphates and pesticides. Deficiency of which, can lead to overstimulation of these receptor sites inducing paralysis of the diaphragm of the lungs and muscular system, convulsions, and/or cardiac arrest.[cxiii]

viii. AChE works by breaking ACh into choline and acetic acid. These reactions are necessary to allow a cholinergic activated neuron or muscle to return to its resting state after deactivation. Deficiency of AChE leads to retained activation of the ACh receptor sites: causing excessive salivation and eye-watering in low doses, followed by muscle spasms, paralysis, and ultimately death.[cxiv]

ix. Glyphosate and vaccine induced alterations in the copper/zinc ratio by effecting AChE activity in the brain leads to over occupation of the acetylcholine receptor sites.[cxv]

x. Sperm motility is dependent upon the activation of the nicotinic acetylcholine receptor sites (nAChRs) and the cAMP pathways Glyphosate toxicity reduces the number of and immobilizes sperm by interfering with calcitonin and its regulation of these sites. Glyphosate also interferes with mitochondrial function in sperm resulting in male sterility.[cxvi]

xi. The development of the neural tube, neurulation, in fetuses is dependent upon vitamins cobalamin (B12) and folate (B9). This process of primary neurulation is conserved across all species such as amphibians, reptiles, birds, and mammals. Neurulation is a self-initiating reflex of DNA expression that is critically self-regulated by the DNA, systemic pH levels, and the signaling action of various enzymatic proteins. Glyphosate causes neural tube defects, microcephaly, and birth defects due to a deficiency in cobalamin (B12) and folate (B9).[cxvii]

> **Glyphosate toxicity has the potential to destroy all living reptile, avian, and mammalian species inhabiting the planet by interfering with the neurulation process. Certainly, all those that live in proximity to exposure and in the streams of water runoff are affected.**

xii. Glyphosate reduces secretion of oxytocin from the pituitary gland and progesterone from luteal cells which can lead to the impairment of fertilization, deregulation of uterine contractions, or failure to maintain gestation.[cxviii] It reduces the maternal instincts of love, nurturing and care for the infant, and the ability to orgasm.

xiii. Glyphosate (and heavy metals) inhibit aromatase, the enzyme that facilitates the conversion of androgens to estrogens. Placental estrogens normally help mature brain myelin sheaths, the corpus callosum, and preferentially the left hemisphere of the brain. Glyphosate toxicity inhibits the aromatase conversion of androgens constricting brain blood vessels, elevating brain serotonin, and reducing oxytocin levels. Glyphosate-induced estrogen depletion coherently explains white matter asymmetry, low brain blood flow, hyperexcitability, and social anxiety, more especially in autistic males. Insufficient maternal oxytocin at birth limits fetal brain chloride/water balance and depletes GABA concentrations leading to hyperactivity.[cxix]

Comments: Samuel Hahnemann, the German physician who articulated homeopathy, defines health in the following way:

> **'In the healthy condition of Man, the spiritual vital force (autocracy), the dynamis that animates the material body (organism), rules with unbounded sway, and retains all the parts of the organism in admirable, harmonious, vital operation, as regards both sensations and functions, so that our indwelling, reason-gifted mind can freely employ this**

living, healthy instrument for the higher purpose of our existence.'[cxx]

In accordance to the blueprint encoded into laws of nature, critical regulation of neurotransmitters and hormones in humans and animals gives correct experience, perception, and reactive responses to the world we live in. Our bodies grow and mature from the point of conception into fully functioning vital organisms that have subjective and objective experiences of the world. Consciousness is the awareness of the living being inside the physiological machinery: the awareness of a being which is connected to all things whose body is equipped with receptor sites designed to experience the unified field of this physical reality. Harmony experienced is the result of a perfect and sublime internal balance and a relationship maintained between the viruses and bacteria in our body, the nutrition of the food we eat, the external environment within which we live, and the neurotransmitter and hormone regulation of our physical, neurological, and emotional systems.

Conscience is the awareness of the possibility of transgression in thought or deed that works against our own psyche, our fellow man, and/or the planet that sustains us. Compassion and forgiveness are the vehicles by which we redeem ourselves and remember who we are. Freedom is the ability to realize our full potential as a direct expression of Creation. Consciousness, and living according to our conscience, allows us to experience, through our vagus nerve, the love that exists all around us, not as an abstract projection of our will, but as a surrender to the gravitational system that holds our physical body and emotional sensitivity in time and space.

As humans we are gifted free will to live in accordance to nature's laws or not. However, perverted will and errors of thinking will subvert the vital physiological functions of the body, mind, and emotions. Wrong thinking, based on ego driven desires and aversions (fear, lack, greed, anger, pleasure, etc.), detract from the awareness of ourselves as sentient beings and result in pain and suffering.

This pain and suffering IS the built in self-corrective mechanism of wrong thinking designed to protect our sovereignty and to keep us working in alignment with nature's laws.

Conversely, toxicity driven alterations in our physical chemistry can pervert ones' perception and desires. Toxicological disfunction in any aspect of the subtle chemical interactions of our living, twists and distorts the grace of Man, his understanding, thoughts, and deeds.

From the honorable statesmen to the homeless on the streets, from artistic masters to military masterminds, from the giving mother to the drug addict child, we are all subject to and susceptible to alterations and dysregulation. For in the one there is love and connection to the natural order and in the other, there is hatred, disconnect, and corruption of that same order.

The physiological roots of glyphosate dysregulation are bacterial deficiencies leading to nutritional deficiencies, and the subsequent dysregulation of hormones, neurotransmitters, or receptor sites which register, or don't, the transferences in communication pathways. The psychological or ego driven roots of the sickness that drives the justification for crippling the food chain, and the entire planet, with glyphosate, is a condition that needs a profound rectification between our comprehension of who we really are in relation to the biosphere that makes this all possible. Ignorance of the facts does not preclude us from suffering the consequences.

This glyphosate dysregulation creates an experience of life mutated to the point of unrecognition of ourselves and the world around us. Lost is any sense of the unified field, love, GOD, or connection to nature. Rather, the human race is becoming infertile, depressed, violent, illogical, disconnected, suffering from neurological conditions, developmental delays, cancer, and a host of other progressive degenerative diseases.

Simultaneously we are lost at war, suffer under the tyranny of political corruption, and participate in capitalistic economic systems that are driving destruction of the environment for the sake of what? There are increasing levels of poverty, homelessness, and mental sickness, incapacitating entire communities and nations. There are individuals paralyzed from their self-abuse with tobacco, drug, and food addictions: individuals blindly consuming the products that are harming

them and perpetuating the world trade franchises and multinationals in the supply chain that are poisoning the farmers that produce these very same products.

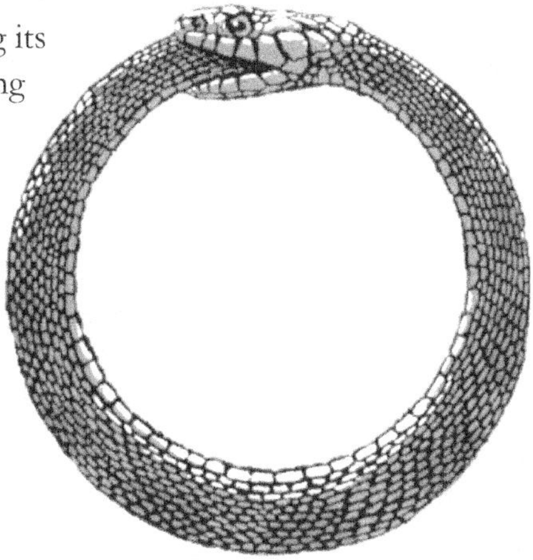

Symbolic of this is the snake eating its own tail, the Ouroboros. Reminding us that which is within us is also outside us and cannot be separate nor extinguished.

Strung out like this, we rely upon consumerism, junk food, fake news, pharmaceutical or recreational drugs to try to resurrect some semblance of balance within ourselves.

We are addicted to faulty systems of government, food, and medicines that are making us sicker, driven by a callous disregard for the environment and our fellow man. It is all based on the lies we have told ourselves about who we are and why we are here. Where there once was order there is now disorder. Where there once was beauty, we now live amidst our ruin.

As physical beings we have lost our way and nature is crying out for us to do something. The animals are crying out. Our bodies are crying out. Our children are crying out. What can be done?

In health, by our very nature, the living human being (body, mind, and soul) must be seen, valued, praised, known, heard, and listened to. We succumb to disease when we are laughed at, ignored, insulted, misunderstood, devalued, and disregarded. In the first there is expansion of the individual and in the second there is contraction. In the first there is becoming and feeling, in the second there is numbing and incapacitation. The living breathing earth responds in this same way. Where we show gratitude and respect, nature flourishes; where we dump our trash and neglect, wastelands prevail.

What injury has been inflicted upon the individual and collective Man that has led him to such abuses of himself, each other, the planet? What injury in his psyche has led to the denial of his very own existence as a pure expression of the **Generating-Organizing-Delivering/Destroying system** of the unified field? If we each can address this conflict within ourselves, then, and only then, can we come to know our pure essence and live at peace with our physical bodies and the elemental forces that mirror us.

Only then will we be able to live in accordance to our conscience and actively connect to the pure vital force of the universe. When we live in accordance to 'Ahimsa,' the Hindu philosophy of respect for all living things and avoidance of violence toward others, then we can experience our own self-healing, self-editing, and self-correcting capacity. When we accurately see and are at peace with what we are, spontaneously we will connect to all.

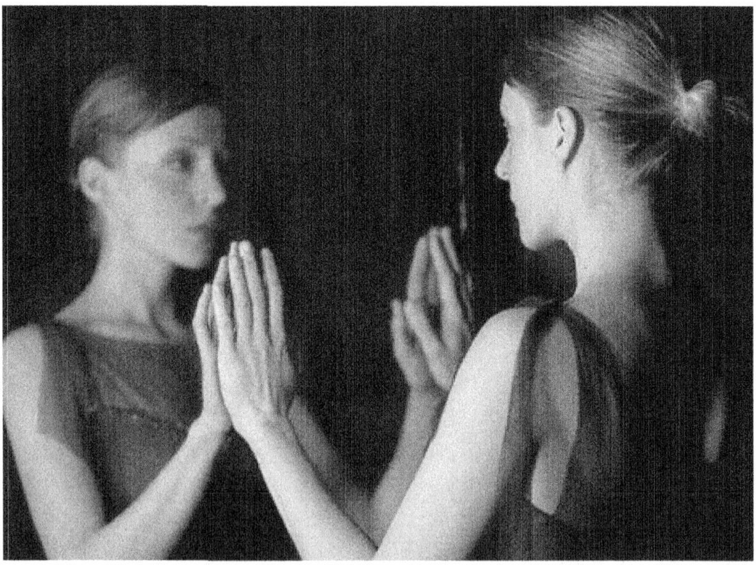

cix Yassine Ait Bali, Saadia Ba-Mhamed, and Mohamed Bennis. Behavioral and Immunohistochemical Study of the Effects of Subchronic and Chronic Exposure to Glyphosate in Mice. Frontiers in Behavioral Neuroscience. 2017; 11: 146. https://www.ncbi.nlm.nih.gov/pmc/articles/PMC5550406/.

cx Anthony Samsel and Stephanie Seneff. Glyphosate, pathways to modern diseases III: Manganese, neurological diseases, and associated pathologies. Surg Neurol Int. 2015; 6: 45. https://www.ncbi.nlm.nih.gov/pmc/articles/PMC4392553/.

cxi Ibid.

cxii Ibid.

cxiii Glusczak L, dos Santos Miron D, Crestani M, Braga da Fonseca M, de Araújo Pedron F, Duarte MF, Vieira VL. Effect of glyphosate herbicide on acetylcholinesterase activity and metabolic and hematological parameters in piava (Leporinus obtusidens). Ecotoxicol Environ Saf. 2006 Oct;65(2):237-41. https://www.ncbi.nlm.nih.gov/pubmed/16174533.

cxiv Anthony Samsel and Stephanie Seneff. Glyphosate, pathways to modern diseases IV: cancer and related pathologies. Journal of Biological Physics and Chemistry 15(3):121-159. January 2015. https://www.researchgate.net/publication/283490944_Glyphosate_pathways_to_modern_diseases_IV_cancer_and_related_pathologies.

cxv Fatemeh Sayehmiri, MSc, Nasim Babaknejad, MSc, Somayeh Bahrami, MSc, Kourosh Sayehmiri, PhD, Mojtaba Darabi, MD ,1 and Mostafa Rezaei-Tavirani, PhD. Zn/Cu Levels in the Field of Autism Disorders: A Systematic Review and Meta-analysis. Iran J Child Neurol. 2015 Autumn; 9(4): 1–9. https://www.ncbi.nlm.nih.gov/pmc/articles/PMC4670971/.

cxvi George Anifandis, George Amiridis, Konstantinos Dafopoulos, Alexandros Daponte, Eleni Dovolou, Eleftherios Gavriil, Vyron Gorgogietas, Elli Kachpani, Zissis Mamuris, Christina I. Messini, Katerina Vassiou, Anna-Maria G. Psarra. The In Vitro Impact of the Herbicide Roundup on Human Sperm Motility and Sperm

Mitochondria. Toxics. 2018 Mar; 6(1): 2. https://www.ncbi.nlm.nih.gov/pmc/articles/PMC5874775/.

cxvii Anthony Samsel and Stephanie Seneff. Glyphosate, pathways to modern diseases II: Celiac sprue and gluten intolerance. Interdiscip Toxicol. 2013 Dec. https://www.ncbi.nlm.nih.gov/pmc/articles/PMC3945755/.

cxviii Wrobel, MH. Glyphosate affects the secretion of regulators of uterine contractions in cows while it does not directly impair the motoric function of myometrium in vitro. Toxicol Appl Pharmacol. 2018 Jun 15;349:55-61. https://www.ncbi.nlm.nih.gov/pubmed/29705296.

cxix Good, P. Evidence the U.S. autism epidemic initiated by acetaminophen (Tylenol) is aggravated by oral antibiotic amoxicillin/clavulanate (Augmentin) and now exponentially by herbicide glyphosate (Roundup). Clinical Nutrition ESPEN. 2018 Feb;23:171-183. https://www.ncbi.nlm.nih.gov/pubmed/29460795.

cxx Hahnemann, Samuel. Organon of Medicine. Paragraph 9. Dec.1921. Online version. The School of Homeopathy. https://www.homeopathyschool.com/the-school/editorial/the-organon/aphorism-1-10/.

8. Clinical Conditions of Glyphosate Toxicity

- ADD, ADHD, OCD, autism.
- Allergies, asthma.
- Alzheimer's disease.
- Anemia. Night sweats.
- Birth defects.
- Broken hair and nails, collagen malformation, twisting or pulling of the spine, tendons, and ligaments.
- Celiac and gluten intolerance. Bloating, inability to digest food, wheat intolerance. Absorption and deficiency issues.
- Colitis, constipation.
- Depression, suicidal thoughts, apathy.
- Enzymatic dysfunction.
- Environmental sensitivities.
- Endocrine dysregulation, thyroid dysfunction, hyper- and hypothyroidism, infertility. Low progesterone levels, increased miscarriages. Neonatal developmental deficiencies.
- Headaches like a vise: especially from wine or beer.
- Histamine reactions. Excess histamine causing chronic inflammation. Mast cell activation disease.
- Improper metabolism of nitrogen in purines and uric acid: leads to gout, urticaria, hives, allergic conditions, skin lesions, and eczema. Itching without eruptions. Weeping dermatitis.
- Lactic acidosis, cerebral inflammation.
- Kidney disease. Gout, Nephritis, Hypertension, Diabetes.
- Leukemia and other cancers.
- Obesity, water retention, systemic inflammation.
- *Candida* overgrowth. Brain fog, bloating, fermented stools.
- Other symptoms and conditions not yet documented.

Sourced. [cxxi, cxxii]

1. **Celiac Disease**: Inability to digest wheat and gluten. Symptoms include nausea, diarrhea, skin rashes, macrocytic anemia, and depression. It is a multifactorial disease associated with numerous nutritional deficiencies as well as reproductive issues and increased risk to thyroid disease, kidney failure, and cancer.

Corresponding increase in Celiac Disease compared to increases in Glyphosate usage. [cxxiii]

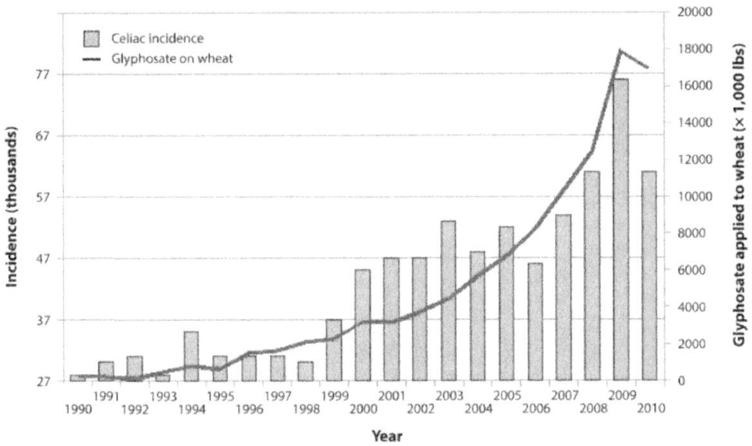

2. **Disturbance in Healthy Intestinal Biome**: Leading to leaky gut syndrome, and populations of other harmful bacteria and/or *Candida* over-growth.
3. **Elevated Histamine Levels**: This can be from the excess lactic acid and uric acid due to incomplete purine reduction, from allergic reaction to lacto-fermenting bacteria or excess lactic acid due to insufficient molybdenum dependent enzymes that convert lactic acid to lactate, which serves to normalize pH and can be used in cells for energy. Histamine is also a protein dependent on diamine oxidase (DAO)(copper inhibiting and zinc dependent) for oxidation (to reduce histamine levels). Diamine oxidase transcription is glycine dependent.
4. **Cytochrome P450 (CYP) Driven Enzyme Impairment and Sulfate Depletion**: CYP's are a class of glycine dependent hemoproteins (Fe^{+4} base) that act as substrates for enzymatic function in vertebrates. CYP proteins are vital for the creation of

bile acids, activation of vitamin D, detoxification of heavy metals and drugs, and normal metabolism. Substitution of glyphosate instead of glycine causes a malfunction of CYP proteins leading to damage of the liver and kidneys due to failure of metabolic detoxification pathways (glutathione). Impairment of these proteins leads to a reduction in the creation of bile acids and resultant elevated blood cholesterol, pancreatitis, and early death. Bile acids are conjugated with taurine or glycine in the liver, and further conjugated with sodium or potassium salts to form bile salts. Primary bile acids are those synthesized by the liver from circulating cholesterol. Secondary bile acids result from commensal bacterial actions in the intestines. Glycine deficiency does not allow for the creation of bile acids in the liver, resulting in elevated blood cholesterol levels. CYP P450 proteins are also vitally important in the production of the steroids and sex hormones produced in the adrenal cortex. CYP dependent aromatase enzyme is responsible for the synthesis of estradiol and testosterone. Glyphosate driven disruption of this pathway leads to an impaired ratio of the sex hormones resulting in a variety of hormonal irregularities: infertility, failure to sexually mature, excess or deficient hormone levels, amenorrhea, etc.

5. **Retinoic Acid (Vitamin A), Celiac Disease, and Reproductive Issues**: Glyphosate drives a deficiency of the CYP enzyme needed to break down retinoic acid. Excess retinoic acid increases the risk of Celiac by suppressing transglutaminase activity. Glyphosate is a teratogenic agent that has an impact on embryos such as impairment of hind-brain development and cleft palate. Retinoic acid is an essential nutrient necessary for early perinatal development however, excess has been shown to produce marked alterations in cephalic and neural crest development and shortening of the anterior-posterior (A-P) axis. These alterations on neural crest markers are correlated with deformities in the cranial cartilages, including a gradual loss of rhombomere domains, reduction of the optic vesicles, and microcephaly.[cxxiv] Infertility can arise from retinoic acid driven abnormalities in sperm morphology along with endocrine dysfunction.

6. **Cobalamin Deficiency**: Cobalamin is Vitamin B12. Those with Celiac disease have elevated levels of homocysteine which is associated with folate (B9) and cobalamin (B12) deficiency. Destabilizations of *Bifidobacteria*, which biosynthesizes cobalamin (B12) and folate (B9), creates a deficiency in both which are crucial for perinatal development, the synthesis and repair of DNA, and creation of neurotransmitters.
7. **Anemia and Iron (Fe) Deficiency**: Glyphosate interferes with iron assimilation in plants and in humans. Glyphosate acts as a chelator of iron and pulls it out through the urine. Depletion in iron leads to depletion in CYP iron dependent hemoproteins. In addition, iron is needed to activate the enzyme xanthine oxidase which oxidizes xanthine to uric acid. Deficient iron leads to a host of immune system challenges, reduction in hemoglobin and erythropoietin which is necessary for red blood cell production. *Candida* overgrowth, from glyphosate induced gut dysbiosis, also adds to iron deficiency.
8. **Molybdenum (Mo) Deficiency**: Celiac disease, or gluten intolerance, leads to a molybdenum deficiency. Molybdenum is essential for the enzymes sulfite oxidase and xanthine oxidase, which are responsible for the conversions of sulfite to sulphate in protein metabolism, and the production of uric acid from hypoxanthine oxidation, respectively. Molybdenum is also essential for purine metabolism. Sulphate is necessary for the creation of the extracellular matrices of all cell types. A healthy methylation cycle is also dependent on Molybdenum. Hyper-lactic-acidosis is also linked to molybdenum deficiency. A hyper-acidic system will create an environment suitable for candida overgrowth, elevated histamine, and changes the functionality of other enzymes. Molybdenum deficiency is also responsible for adenosine deaminase (ADA) deficiency and can lead to inflammatory immune conditions driven by excess adenosine or alterations in RNA gene editing. Heavy metals, excess copper, or silver inhibit the action of ADA.
9. **Manganese (Mn) Deficiency**: Glyphosate inhibits a plant's uptake of manganese needed for photosynthesis. *Lactobacillus* depend critically on Mn for antioxidant protection. Reduced

intestinal *Lactobacillus* leads to overgrowth of the pathogen *Salmonella*, which is resistant to glyphosate toxicity. Gut dysbiosis, depression, anxiety, Parkinson's disease (PD), and prion disease can all result from manganese (Mn) deficiency. Sperm motility depends on Mn, and this may partially explain increased rates of infertility and birth defects.[cxxv] Mn is important to the enzyme glutamine synthetase (GS) that converts glutamate to L-glutamine making the glutamate harmless. GS is preferentially activated by magnesium, but manganese, cobalt, and iron will also work. GS is present predominantly in the brain, kidneys, and liver. GS in the brain participates in the metabolic regulation of glutamate, the detoxification of brain ammonia, the assimilation of ammonia, recyclization of neurotransmitters, and termination of neurotransmitter signals. GS in the brain is found primarily in astrocytes. Astrocytes protect neurons against excitotoxicity by taking up excess ammonia and glutamate. Excess glutamate in the brain leads to hyperactivity.

10. **Selenium (Se) and Thyroid Disorders**: Healthy thyroid function is dependent upon selenium, iron, zinc, and iodine. Glyphosate disrupts selenium uptake in plants so plants become deficient in selenium. *Lactobacillus* convert inorganic selenium to the organic forms selenocysteine and selenomethionine. Selenium deficiency impairs thyroid hormone metabolism by inhibiting the synthesis and activity of the iodothyronine deiodinase, which converts Thyroxine (T4) to the more metabolically active 3,3',5-triiodothyronine (T3). Iron deficiency impairs thyroid hormone synthesis by reducing activity of CYP heme-dependent thyroid peroxidase. A deficiency in selenium will also result in an iodine deficiency. Selenium helps protect against iodine toxicity by ensuring that glutathione peroxidase activity in the thyroid is adequate. Correct iodine levels are key to perinatal development.
11. **Indole and Kidney Disease**: Indole is biosynthesized in the shikimate-acid pathway of commensal bacteria. It is an intermediate in the biosynthesis of Tryptophan. Disruption of EPSP synthase and failure to synthesize tryptophan leads to excess of indole. Indole is also a product of *Clostridia*l and *E. coli* species, the presence of which leads to heightened intestinal inflammation.

Indole acts as an intercellular signaling molecule. It regulates various aspects of bacterial physiology, including spore formation, plasmid stability, resistance to drugs, biofilm formation, and virulence. However, glyphosate driven reduction in healthy intestinal bacteria and increases in pathogenic bacteria which raises indole concentrations. This promotes inflammation of the intestinal lining, leading to Celiac disease, which begins the release of other inflammatory cytokines that damage kidney cells. Indole also inhibits the growth of cobalamin-producing microorganisms which can lead to pernicious anemia.

12. **Nutritional Deficiencies**: Due to disruption of the gut biome, which is responsible for enzymes and digestive process. This also leads to inflammation in the intestinal wall impairing nutritional absorption. Glyphosate interrupts the *Bifidobacteria* dependent biosynthesis of B vitamins that include thiamine (B1), riboflavin (B2), niacin (B3), pantothenic acid (B5), pyridoxine (B6), biotin (B7), folate (B9), and cobalamin (B12). Vitamin B3, niacin, is a necessary constituent of NAD (nicotinamide adenine dinucleotide), a co-enzyme necessary for all protein metabolism; cobalamin (B12) is needed for DNA synthesis and the metabolism of fatty acids and proteins. Folate (B9) is necessary for iron absorption and neural tube development.
13. **Endocrine Disruption**: Glyphosate is an endocrine disruptor in human cells.[cxxvi] It causes the multiplication of estrogen sensitive human breast cancer cells.[cxxvii] An endocrine disruptor is a chemical that either mimics or blocks hormones and disrupts the body's normal functions. This disruption can happen through altering normal hormone levels, halting or stimulating the production of excess hormones, or interacting directly with the organ the hormone was meant to regulate.[cxxviii] Endocrine disruptors can increase or decrease hormone production, imitate hormones or even transform one hormone into another. Endocrine disruptors can also tell cells to die prematurely, compete with essential nutrients, and build up in hormone-producing organs. These imbalances and malfunctions of the endocrine system can lead to diabetes, hypertension, obesity, kidney disease, cancer (breast, prostate, liver, brain, thyroid, non-Hodgkin's lymphoma);[cxxix,cxxx]

Osteoporosis, Cushing's syndrome, hypo- and hyperthyroidism, infertility, birth defects, erectile dysfunction;[cxxxi] sexual maturity problems and neurological disorders such as: learning disabilities, attention deficit disorder (ADD);[cxxxii] autism;[cxxxiii] dementia;[cxxxiv] Alzheimer's;[cxxxv] Parkinson's, and schizophrenia.[cxxxvi] Endocrine disruptors are especially damaging to organisms undergoing hormonal changes: fetuses, babies, children, adolescents, and the elderly.

14. **Cancer**: Increased oxidative stress due to lack of essential enzymes necessary to remove oxalates leads to increased genetic mutation and failure for reproducing cells to differentiate. Antioxidants are primary in preventing cancer. Glutathione is one such antioxidant that serves to oxidize oxalates. Cancer is a result of this, primarily T cell leukemia, but other cancers can also develop.

Neural Tube Defects: Summary of Clinical Findings Possibly Related to Agricultural Chemicals on the Palouse[cxxxvii]

Contribution by Kelly Zakariasen. "I live and practice homeopathy in a small community, Moscow, Idaho, which sits in the heart of a region known as the "Palouse." It has been termed the "Tuscany of the West" and is a large agricultural area for wheat, canola, and legumes. Most are grown conventionally and are heavily sprayed. Because of the flat landscape, crop dusting is very common.

"Our family moved here from Ely, Minnesota nearly eight years ago and I began a limited homeopathic practice in 2013. My current clientele are mostly women of childbearing age and their children.

"Over time I began to hear of frequent and recurrent miscarriages and also had clients who experienced these symptoms. An online survey of 100 women, conducted by myself and one of my clients, found the recurrent miscarriage rate among women ages 18-29 to be 27%, ages 30-39 was 33%, and ages 40-49 was 45%. I contacted Washington State University in nearby Pullman, WA to inquire as to whether they had ever conducted a study on pregnancy loss (they had not and had no plans to). I spoke with several local midwives who have seen a higher than the national average rate of miscarriage. In my small sampling of clients, I document the following in my own clinical practice:"

The below charted findings from 2015, suggest the deleterious effects of environmental exposure to glyphosate on endocrine function, B12 and folate (B9) deficiencies, and the neurulation process in utero. International miscarriage rates are normally 15-20%.[cxxxviii]

Pregnancy and Miscarriage Comparison. Moscow, Idaho (2015).		
Complaint	Incidence	Comments
Unexplained Infertility	22%	Client's ages between 20-29.
Pregnancy Loss (1)	66%	Generally, before 12 weeks gestation.
Recurrent Pregnancy Loss (2+)	50%	One client had experienced 5 losses, usually in the second trimester. She had 3 living children.
Premature Birth	22%	Average gestation 32-34 weeks; one client came having had 3 pregnancies with oligohydramnios (deficiency of amniotic fluid).
Birth Defects	11%	Velamentous cord insertion, intrauterine growth restriction, spina bifida.
Allergies	50%	Seasonal allergies (hay fever, spring and fall during planting and harvest time, allergies to wool, and dust, eczema).

The chart below from January 2019, suggests an escalation of miscarriage rates in this region from 2015 to 2019.[cxxxix]

Pregnancy and Miscarriage Comparison. Moscow, Idaho (2019).										
# of respondents	23	# of pregnancies	23	Live births	7	# of losses	16			
Age of respondents	18-24	25-34	35-44	45-54						
	1	15	5	2						
Age groups for losses	18-29	30-39	40-49							
# of pregnancy losses	12	3	1							
# of second pregnancy losses	4	1								
# of pregnancies per person	1	2	3	4	5	6	7	8	9	10
	2	0	6	6	2	1	4	1	0	1
Total # of losses	1	2	3	4	5					
	11	3	0	1	1					
Gestational age of loss in weeks	4-6	7-9	10-12							
	10	4	2							
69.6% of all pregnancies miscarried.										
75% of losses were in the prime reproductive period ages 18-29 years.										
31.3 % had multiple losses.										
62.5% of pregnancy losses were during weeks 4-6, the time of neurulation. Vitamin B12 and folate (B9) dependent.										

cxxi Anthony Samsel and Stephanie Seneff. Glyphosate, pathways to modern diseases II: Celiac sprue and gluten intolerance. Interdiscip Toxicol. 2013 Dec. https://www.ncbi.nlm.nih.gov/pmc/articles/PMC3945755/.

cxxii Seneff, Stephanie. Multiple articles and research on glyphosate, autism, obesity, Celiac disease and more. http://people.csail.mit.edu/seneff/.

cxxiii Ibid.

cxxiv Paganelli A, Gnazzo V, Acosta H, López SL, Carrasco AE. Glyphosate-based herbicides produce teratogenic effects on vertebrates by impairing retinoic acid signaling. Chem Res Toxicol. 2010 Oct 18;23(10):1586-95. https://www.ncbi.nlm.nih.gov/pubmed/20695457.

cxxv Anthony Samsel and Stephanie Seneff. Glyphosate, pathways to modern diseases III: Manganese, neurological diseases, and associated pathologies. Surg Neurol Int. 2015; 6: 45. https://www.ncbi.nlm.nih.gov/pmc/articles/PMC4392553/.

cxxvi Gasnier, C., Dumont, C., Benachour, N., Clair, E., Chagnon, M.C. and Séralini, G.E. Glyphosate-based herbicides are toxic and endocrine disruptors in human cell lines. Toxicology, 262(3): 184-191, 2009.

cxxvii Thongprakaisang, S., Thiantanawat, A., Rangkadilok, N., Suriyo, T. and Satayavivad, J. Glyphosate induces human breast cancer cells growth via estrogen receptors, Food and Chemical Toxicology, 59: 129-136. 2013.

cxxviii Nancy L. Swanson, Andre Leu, Jon Abrahamson. and Bradley Wallet. Genetically engineered crops, glyphosate and the deterioration of health in the United States of America. Journal of Organic Systems, 9(2), 2014. https://jeffreydachmd.com/wp-content/uploads/2015/04/Genetically-engineered-crops-glyphosate-deterioration-health-United-States-Swanson-J-Organic-Systems-20141.pdf.

cxxix Ibid.

cxxx Marc, J., Mulner-Lorillon, O. and Bellé, R. Glyphosate-based pesticides affect cell cycle regulation, Biology of the Cell, 96(3): 245-249. 2004.

cxxxi Soto, A.M. and Sonnenschein, C. Environmental causes of cancer: endocrine disruptors as carcinogens, Nature Reviews Endocrinology. 6: 363-370. 2010.

cxxxii de Cock, M., Maas, Y.G., and Van de Bor, M. Does perinatal exposure to endocrine disruptors induce autism spectrum and attention deficit hyperactivity disorders? Acta Pediatric, 101(8): 811-819, 2012.

cxxxiii Schulkin, J. Autism and the amygdala: An endocrine hypothesis. Brain and Cognition, 65(1): 87-99. 2007.

cxxxiv Ghosh, A. Endocrine, metabolic, nutritional, and toxic disorders leading to dementia. Annals of Indian Academy of Neurology, (Suppl 2): S63-8. 2010.

cxxxv Merlo, S., Spampinato, S., Canonico, P.L., Copani, A. and Sortino, M.A. Alzheimer's disease: brain expression of a metabolic disorder? Trends in Endocrinology and Metabolism, 21(9): 537- 544. 2010.

cxxxvi MacSweeney, D., Timms, P. and Johnson, A. Preliminary communication thyro-endocrine pathology, obstetric morbidity and schizophrenia: survey of a hundred families with a schizophrenic proband. Psychological Medicine, 8(1): 151-155. 1978.

cxxxvii Zakariasen, Kelly. Summary of Clinical Findings of Miscarriage Possibly Related to Agricultural Chemicals on the Palouse. Moscow, Idaho. April 2015. kelly@ajoyfulhearthealth.com.

cxxxviii Diane M Fraser and Margaret A Cooper. Myles Textbook for Midwives. 15th Edition. Churchill Livingston's Elsevier. UK. 2009. Pg. 314.

cxxxix Zakariasen, Kelly. Summary of Clinical Findings of Miscarriage Possibly Related to Agricultural Chemicals on the Palouse. Moscow, Idaho. January 2019. kelly@ajoyfulhearthealth.com.

9. Summary: Absorption Routes and Complications of Glyphosate

Glyphosate is used on the plants we eat in combination with detergents that make the plant cell membranes and walls more permeable to uptake the water soluble glyphosate. After glyphosate has penetrated the plant cells it interferes with all enzymatic action that takes place in those cells, limiting the uptake of vital nutrients and mitochondrial function, it gets incorporated into the DNA and RNA strands of those plants. As plants enter the food chain and we, or animals (which then we consume) eat glyphosate-contaminated plants the entire food chain is destroyed. The added detergents in glyphosate products facilitates the crossover of glyphosate through cell membranes. This disrupts not only our cellular activity, but that of all other living things in the food chain: bacteria, worms, sperm, frogs, mice, birds, possums, fish, cats dogs, cows, deer, whales, etc.

The roman numerals assigned to the following issues correspond to the identically numerated items in chapter **14. Homeopathic Remedies to Repair Glyphosate Damage**.

I. Biome and Intestinal Lining:

Glyphosate that is consumed in the foods we eat first kills the commensal bacteria and the tight junction gating ability in our digestive track. This then interferes with the digestive and inflammatory processes as a significant number of precursory amino acids, and digestive enzymes. The immunological regulatory processes starts with a healthy gut biome. All neurotransmitters are dependent upon tryptophan which is synthesized by intestinal bacteria. Previous use of antibiotics at any time in life compounds dysbiosis leading to greater risk of toxicity with glyphosate. The resultant interference of glyphosate in myosin action and gut motility causes constipation and decreased serotonin. Previous vaccination with measles or inactivated polio vaccines (IPV) increases gastrointestinal inflammation or deregulation of the tight junctions respectively. As glyphosate interferes with metabolic processes and ATP production a more acidic intestinal environment is encouraged. This in turn limits the propagation of lacto-fermenting bacteria while encouraging yeast proliferation. The result of low oxygen and yeast overgrowth compounds lactic acidosis. The following bacterial species are encouraged in the presence of glyphosate toxicity and antibiotic resistance.

a. ***Escherichia coli***: Most *E. coli* species are beneficial to the digestive process, metabolizing simple sugars, carbohydrates, and synthesizing proteins. Some species however produce a number of *Shigella*-like toxins that are detrimental and can produce inflammation and cell death of the lining of the intestines, resulting in diarrhea, dysentery, fever, nausea, vomiting, stomach cramps, flatulence, or the auto-immune condition of hemolytic-uremic syndrome.
b. ***Candida albicans***: Produces over 80 chemical toxins capable of making one feel dizzy and fatigued, while shutting down thyroid function, throwing hormones off balance, and causing intense sugar and alcohol cravings and the tendency to gain weight. *Candida* and its by-products are associated with symptoms of PMS, loss of libido, painful intercourse, infertility, numbness, tingling, multiple sclerosis (MS), Crohn's disease, colitis, inflammatory bowel syndrome (IBS), acne, lupus, insomnia, drowsiness, white tongue, bad breath, body odor, sinusitis, bruising, sore throat, bronchitis, shortness of breath, heart palpitations, spots in front of eyes, and dozens more symptoms.
c. ***Clostridia* species**: Leads to neurologically driven intestinal inflammation, inflammatory bowel syndrome (IBS), neurotoxicity by activating acetylcholine receptors in the brain (spasms and paralysis), and tryptophan deficiency resulting in a serotonin deficit increasing pain levels.
d. ***Pseudomonas* variants**: Leads to an increase in formaldehyde and the production of biofilms to protect the bacteria from the immune system in the intestine. These biofilms produce what are called 'rope worms.'
e. ***Salmonella***: Leading to deficiency of the connective tissues, malnutrition, acidosis, inability to digest fats, Celiac disease, vomiting, and hemorrhages.

f. **Tight junction issues**: underdevelopment of the intestinal lining from infancy either caused by antibiotic disruption of the maternal biome, antibiotics given during birth, or being the recipient of the inactivated polio vaccine (IPV) given at two, four, and six months of age, according national vaccine schedules, along with subsequent exposure to glyphosate, wheat or gliadin, drives upregulation of zonulin which opens the tight junctions of the intestinal lining leading to system wide inflammation, elevated histamine and IgE antibody responses, intestinal bloating, and food allergies/ sensitivities.

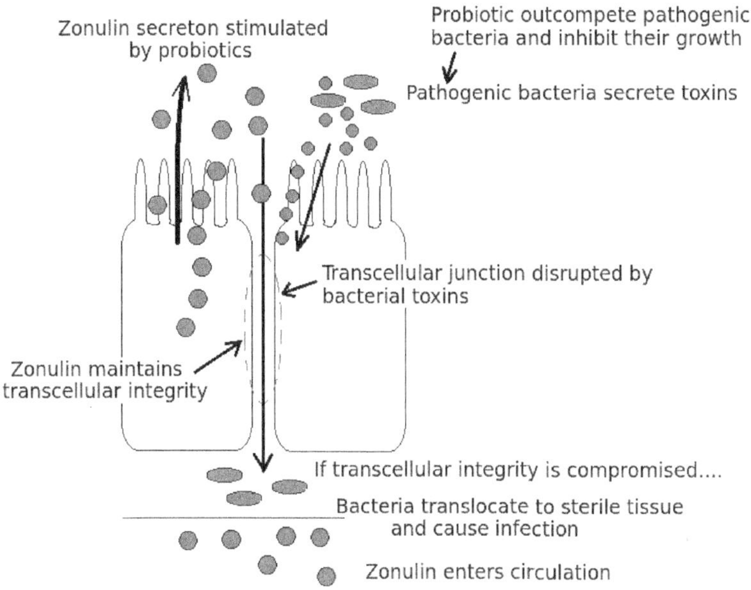

II. Nutritional Deficiencies:

Due to nutritional deficiencies in glyphosate sprayed food and the disturbance of our biomes, further nutritional deficiency or toxicities arise due to imbalances in the ratios of populating bacteria. The main nutrients affected are: sulfur, iron, calcium, manganese, molybdenum, zinc, cobalt, copper, and selenium. With the subsequent lack of enzymes dependent on these essential mineral nutrients all metabolic processes, GPCR receptor site functionality, and disrupts neurotransmitter and hormonal synthesis and regulation. Vitamin D will not be activated in the liver, resulting in deficiency of healthy immune system function. Leaching of calcium leads to the deposit of kidney stones, weakens bones, and interferes with neurotransmitter transmission. Glyphosate also interferes with the calcium ionization of myosin (bowel motility), GPCR site activations (hormone and neurotransmitters receptors), and blood pressure regulation (pituitary gland and vasopressin).

III. Enzymes and Amino Acids:

a. Glyphosate primarily disrupts the RNA synthesis of the following protein enzyme in the shikimate-acid pathway of bacteria by substituting itself in place of glycine: 5-enolpyruvylshikimate-3-phosphate (EPSP) synthase.
b. As a result, this disrupts the creation or functionality of the enzymes pepsin, lipase, trypsin, diamine oxidase (DAO) (copper inhibiting and zinc dependent), and amine oxidase (AO) (copper dependent); amino acid chains that are necessary for starch, protein, and fat digestion, and reduction in histamine production respectively.
c. Other enzymes include glutamate synthase (L-glutamine to glutamate), and glutamine synthetase (NADPH) (glutamate to L-glutamine)(copper and magnesium dependent). Glutamate hydrogenase needed to convert glutamate to urea which is also copper dependent.
d. Tyrosine hydroxylase, thyroid peroxidase, xanthine oxidase, sulfite oxidase, and others.
e. Also glutamic acid decarboxylase (GAD), dependent on the cofactor pyridoxine (B6) along with calcitonin which is essential for the reabsorption of calcium to the bones. Pyridoxine (B6) is normally synthesized by the preferentially killed *Bifidobacteria.*
f. Glyphosate also depletes tyrosine, another amino acid, necessary for proper thyroid function and dopamine production for stable minds.
g. Glyphosate depletes the amino acids tyrosine, tryptophan, and phenylalanine, deficiency of which contributes to changes in all neurotransmitter levels.

h. Deficiencies in CYP hemoprotein (iron) dependent enzymes interferes with hemoglobin production, bile acid and bile salt creation, hormone creation, and thyroid enzyme functionality in the thyroid gland.

IV. Collagen Issues:

Most importantly, glycine is needed for the creation of all collagen which is the main constituent of all fascia and connective tissue in the body. Uptake of glyphosate instead of glycine results in a variety of conditions in the body including weak and deformed collagen, the breakdown of connective tissue, tendons, and ligaments, weak hair and nails, excessive scarring, and in animals, deformities in hoof growth. Glyphosate is stored in the collagen of the body, the omentum of the intestines, and in the liver, until it is released through detoxification. Glyphosate driven hyperthyroidism leads to poor collagen formation and degradation of existing collagen.

V. Liver and Metabolic Issues:

Glyphosate interferes with most every function of the liver. Glyphosate is also stored in the liver and will affect cellular functions and detoxification processes by first interfering with methylation cycles. CYP protein (heme-dependent proteins and enzymes) deficiency leads to bile acid suppression, metabolic issues, detoxification issues, mitochondrial issues, and high cholesterol. Impaired myosin action affects motility of the bile ducts. Reduction in bile acids and bile salts leads to inability to digest and emulsify fats.

VI. Kidneys:

Nephropathy (kidney stones from excess excretion of calcium), nephrolithiasis (formation of kidney stones), elevated uric acid (uremic acidosis), interstitial nephritis (excess cytokines), and hypertension by dysregulation of hypothalamic-pituitary-adrenal axis.

VII. Neurotransmitters, Acetylcholine, and GPCR Sites:

Glyphosate limits lacto-fermenting bacteria vital to neurotransmitter creation and functionality, namely tryptophan, the precursor to phenylalanine, serotonin, glutamate, GABA, dopamine, and melatonin. Deficiency of glycine, necessary for the building and functionality of neurotransmitters, changes outcomes in production and function. Changes in biome upregulates acetylcholine affecting sympathetic and parasympathetic communication along the vagus nerve. Mineral and enzyme deficiencies change functionality of the G-protein coupled receptor sites (GPCRs) changing cholinergic and neurotransmitter signaling. Disruption in neurotransmitter creation and metabolism, receptor activity, regulatory feedback systems and ratios, leads to a host of neurological, physical, psychological, or emotional conditions.

VIII. DNA and RNA:

Glyphosate supplants the normal uptake of glycine which is essential for the creation of the purines needed in to regulate all DNA and RNA replication and transcription. The substitution of glyphosate instead of glycine into the glycine-ring-structures creates inoperable DNA and RNA. As a result, the enzymes and proteins needed for digestion and other vitally important functions in the body, coded for by this DNA, become defective. DNA contamination leads to genetic defects and immune suppression. RNA contamination leads to pathological alterations in the coding of functional proteins thereby affecting the epigenetics of that gene expression.

IX. Endocrine System:

Glyphosate dysregulates the endocrine system with regards to thyroid function, adrenal function, regulation and creation of sex hormones (androgens), blood pressure, and perinatal and childhood brain development by interfering with both the hypothalamic-pituitary-thyroid axis and hypothalamic-pituitary-adrenal axis.

a. **Thyroid Gland**: The thyroid gland regulates metabolic rate and protein synthesis. The amino acid tyrosine is synthesized in the body from the essential amino acid phenylalanine. Phenylalanine must be sourced from food or the bacteria that inhabit the intestines. Tyrosine is a byproduct of the shikimate-acid pathway in both plants and bacteria. The thyroid hormones triiodothyronine (T3) and thyroxine (T4) are created from iodine and tyrosine based on a feed-back loop that stimulates or suppresses the release of thyroid stimulating hormone (TSH) from the anterior pituitary gland. The thyroid also produces the hormone calcitonin, which plays a role in calcium and phosphate homeostasis and thyroid hormone levels.

b. Glyphosate toxicity interferes with the hypothalamic-pituitary-thyroid axis by inducing a phenylalanine deficiency by interrupting the shikimate-acid pathway. As phenylalanine is a precursor of T4, its production is reduced, the result of which can lead to hypothyroidism. Conversely, glyphosate also induces a reduction in the genes encoding the deiodinase enzyme necessary for the conversion of T4 to T3 which can lead to hyperthyroidism. It also interferes with the functionality of the thyroxine (T4) GPCR sites receptive to T4, thus not communicating the excess to the hypothalamus, resulting in continued creation of more thyroid stimulating hormone (TSH), driving hyperthyroidism further. Hypothyroidism can also be induced by manganese deficiency or the impairment of DNA coding for the viability of thyroid stimulating hormone, thus under stimulating the thyroid's creation of thyroxine (T4). Activated EBV also activates auto-immune conditions such as Hashimoto's thyroiditis in the thyroid (starting as hyperthyroidism followed by the auto-immune condition of hypothyroidism) when the immune system develops antibodies against the thyroid to keep thyroxine production in check.

c. **Adrenal Gland**: The adrenal gland is responsible for hormone production in the adrenal cortex. Glyphosate interferes with the hypothalamic-pituitary-adrenal axis responsible for directing levels of adrenocorticotropic hormone (ACTH) aimed at the adrenal medulla for simulating the creation and release of epinephrine (adrenaline).

d. **Androgens**: Glyphosate interferes with the production for the enzyme aromatase, necessary to convert androgens to their end products estrogen, progesterone and testosterone. The creation of these hormones is also dependent on vitamin C. The enzyme G6PD converts vitamin C to a usable form for these reactions. Glyphosate disrupts the functionality of this enzyme thus the conversation of vitamin C. The hypothalamic-pituitary-adrenal axis regulates the creation of hormones from the adrenal cortex; adrenal output of cortisone, adrenaline, and the sex-hormones progesterone, estrogen, and testosterone, which maintain their relative concentrations based on G-protein coupled receptor site functionality in the respective glands and feedback loops to the hypothalamus. Accordingly, all hormonal regulation can be disrupted by lack of any one hormone or receptor site failure. Failure to sexually mature, differentiate ones' sex, infertility, and miscarriage can be a result.

e. **Brain Development**: Glyphosate is responsible for retinoic acid (Vitamin A) deficiency which regulates the CYP protein enzymatic gene signaling of the development of the neural tube. Neurulation is cobalamin (B12) and folate (B9) dependent, as glyphosate depletes these essential vitamins serious defects can arise. It is also responsible for the disruption in the capacity of the pituitary and thyroid to regulate embryonic and fetal development is impaired results in severe birth defects.
f. **Blood Pressure**: Due to the deleterious effects of glyphosate on the kidney's ability to detoxify the body, and disruption of the hormones of the hypothalamic-pituitary-adrenal axis, varying concentrations of vasopressin, modulation in urination output, water retention and/or high blood pressure are a result.
g. **cAMP pathway**: Glyphosate also interferes with the production of cyclic adenosine monophosphate (cAMP). The cAMP-dependent pathway, also known as the adenylyl cyclase enzyme dependent pathway, is a G-protein coupled receptor-triggered signaling cascade used in intracellular communication and responsiveness to hormones in the endocrine system, glucagon levels and sperm motility. Calcitonin is the necessary driver of this signaling pathway.

X. Immune System:

a. Glyphosate driven excess adenosine levels suppresses immune system regulatory functions. Glyphosate causes disruption of the enzyme diamine oxidase (DAO) which reduces histamine levels after allergic reactions, setting up a cascading effect of systemic allergenic responses. This also leads to an over production of IgE antibodies pushing a proliferation of white blood cells resulting in lymphomas or T cell leukemia or a variety of other cancers.

b. Glyphosate driven occupation of the adenosine receptor sites blocks the immune systems' suppression of retroviruses such as human immunodeficiency virus (HIV) virus, Hepatitis B, and further transactivation of these retroviruses by co-infections with herpes viruses such as chickenpox or Epstein-Barr virus, etc., which can lead to shingles or Hashimoto's thyroiditis respectively.

c. Cancer is also a possible outcome due to dysregulation of the immune system and purinergic signaling for DNA transcription, resulting in gene mutations of all cells, not only the cancerous cells but the immune cells that would detect and remove the cancer cells.

d. Glyphosate toxicity confounded with vaccine toxicity sets up a cascade of chronic immunological effects including, but not limited to, hyperproliferation of white blood cells (leukemia), cerebral inflammation, allergies, food sensitivities, asthma, eczema, autism, and more.

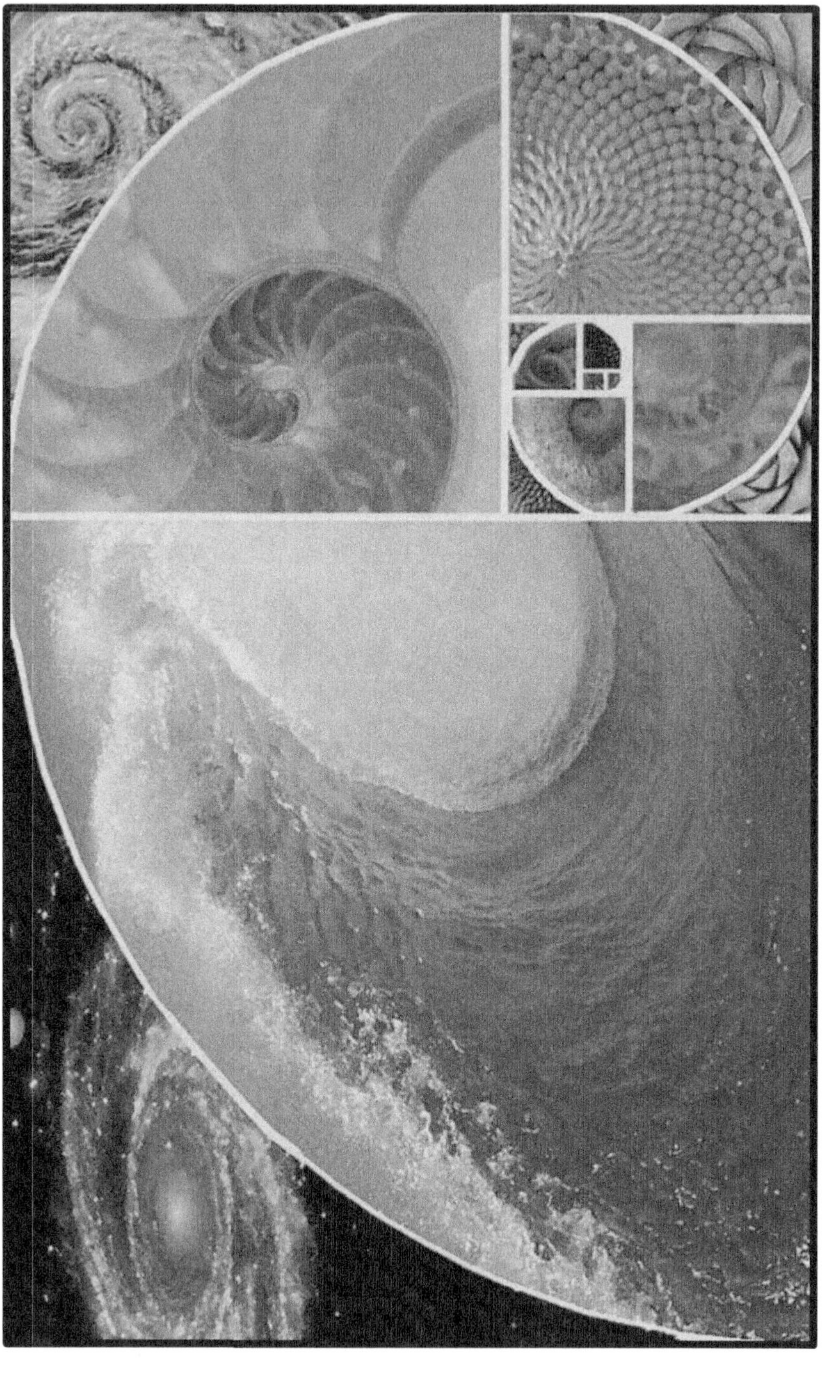

10. Modern Wheat vs Einkorn: Nature's Original Wheat

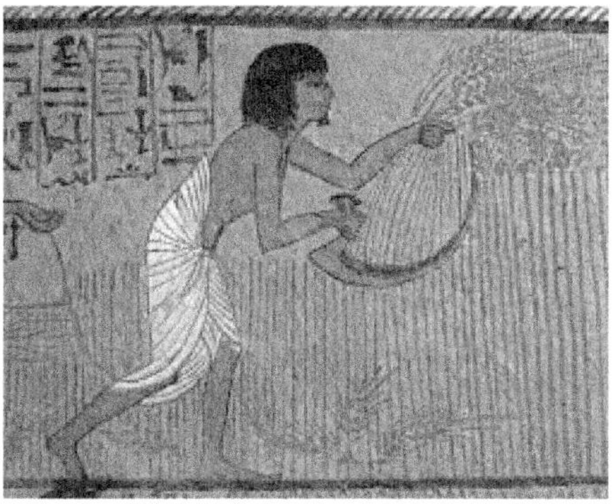

Prior to about 12,000 years ago, in Paleolithic times, Man's earthly existence gradually shifted from hunter gatherer to that of the Neolithic agrarian farmer. To be a hunter gatherer one would always move location based on seasons of plant maturity and the migration patterns of the animal to be eaten. To be a farmer one must stay in one location and work in communities in alignment with the natural rhythm of the sun, seasons and moon cycles in order to ensure healthy crops.

The first wheat to be cultivated by Man was Einkorn wheat (*Triticum monococcum*), a simple diploid grain (two sets of chromosomes), high in protein, manganese, magnesium, iron, thiamine (B1), riboflavin (B2), niacin (B3), and pyridoxine B6. Pyridoxine (B6) serves as a coenzyme in some 100 enzyme reactions in amino acid, glucose, and fat metabolism.

Wheat became known as the staff of life. Indeed, seasonal festivals, mythological stories and religious precedencies were established around planting and harvest times. The moon cycles were acknowledged and honored as they mark off the calendar year that agrarian cultures were bound to. Humans were bound to life in rhythm with nature's cycles. As humans became more successful in an agrarian lifestyle, monetary systems were established with the grain exchange being the foundation upon which all other market values were set.

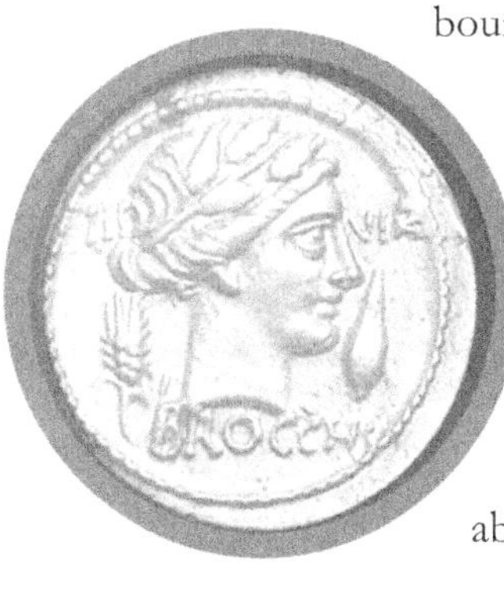

Over time those early farmers abandoned Einkorn wheat for higher yielding varieties, hybridizing and cross cultivating to produce modern wheat. Egalitarian communities became hierarchical with reapers and hoarders, masters and slaves, kings and peasants. Entire banking systems were established upon grain exchange values. Along the way humans came to want, feeling the hunger of poor crops or the psychological entrapment of dependence upon the whim of nature or the masters who took control of this banking system. According to Samuel Hahnemann, in the evolution of Man, this construct was the first instance of disease for humans, that of Psora: the itch and struggle of a static life and scabies which propagated in permanent dwellings.

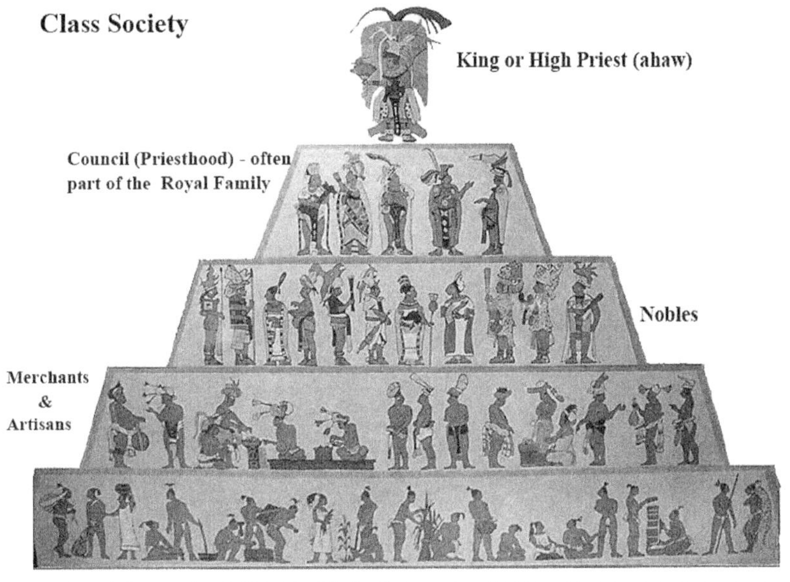

Due to these agrarian practices and the development of living settlements the need for sewer management came about. Polio virus was present in these early populations as an evolutionary measure for the consumption of the newly hybridized wheats. Its purpose was to down regulate zonulin and the tight junctions of the intestinal lining in infancy when the lining was developing so that the child could eat wheat after weening. Passed from human to human through the fecal-oral route, immunity to the virus was conferred from nursing mothers to their infants.

Random historical accounts of polio were documented by the Egyptians and sporadically throughout the ages. However, it never become endemic until increased sanitation measures in the late 19th and mid-20th centuries served to reduce early infant exposure. As they grew to young children, and if they consumed a diet high in wheat, a resultant lack of antibody increased susceptibility to contacting polio.[cxl]

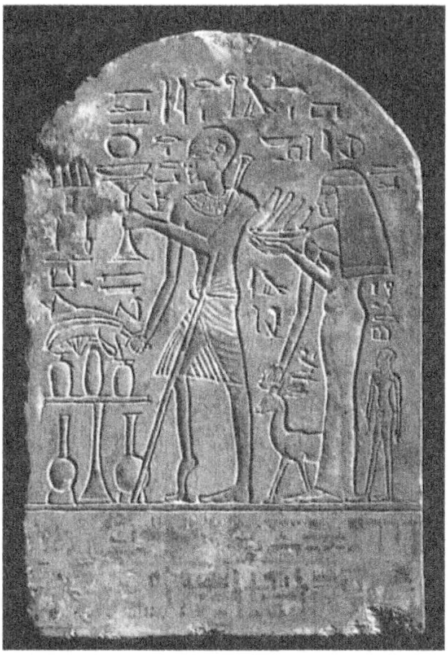

Subsequent exposure to the wild virus in sewer contaminated water brought on polio epidemics worldwide. Without the early down-regulation of the intestinal lining in infancy, the polio virus passes through the gut barrier and enters the nervous system, activating the acetylcholine receptors resulting in paralysis. Open tight junctions activate the sympathetic nervous system into a fight or flight state and allows for fear-based control mechanisms to become more effective. While global polio eradication programs herald themselves for their prophesized eventuality, the co-evolutionary relationship between wheat based agrarian culture and the need for wild polio virus to regulate zonulin has been overlooked.

Commercial wheat, now an eight-chromosome grain due to modern agricultural practices, is virtually nutrient deficient and must be fortified with synthetic nutrients. It has been selected for higher proportion of gliadin variants to glutenin variants. Gliadins facilitate more elasticity of the gluten and the ability to rise during the baking process. The higher gliadin content is causing growing numbers of people to be affected with chronic inflammatory conditions, Celiac disease, leaky gut and leaky brain disorders, obesity, developmental delays and increasing levels of auto-neurotoxicity. The exotoxins released by the body in relation to gluten satiates opioid pain receptors while simultaneously opening the tight junctions, causing fear and paralysis. This cycle leads to greater consumption of wheat or addiction to opioids to numb the pain of that same fear, to numb the pain of the wars activated by global political manipulations.

The only possibility for humanity to reduce these conditions is either total abstinence of wheat, the reintroduction of wild polio virus, or to return to consuming ancient grains like Einkorn. While Einkorn is higher on over all protein content than conventional wheat, an entire group of *y*-gliadins are absent, thus making it more digestible and not interfering with zonulin levels.

Modern agriculture practices with its mono crops, grown on barren soil, artificially propped up by increasing amounts of toxic fertilizers, herbicides, and pesticides, is destroying the environment and life itself. Human beings are now disconnected from the rhythms of nature, and the natural bounty of the earth. Meanwhile, world over, entire governmental and banking systems are on the brink of collapse as a result of capitalistic economies that no longer respect us as individuals or the earth which we depend upon. Rapidly and collectively we are destroying the environment and the entire human race.

On my journey of self-healing, and in service to the planet, I began a search for a homeopathic remedy that would address this disease of 'fear and lack' in humanity that perpetuates pollution of the earth, and the poisoning of our food chain and our children for the sake of profit.

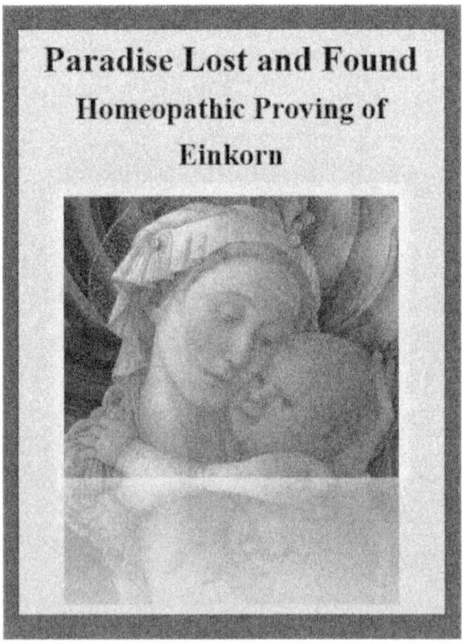

The global vaccination movement, especially by the inactivated polio virus vaccine (IPV), has the same root of fear and profiteering at its base and is at the risk of permanently damaging every child's immune system for the sake of what? So we can eat more of the genetically modified wheat that has been sprayed with glyphosate, inject more vaccines into infants' immune systems, and instigate wars to control the world banking system?

At a conference in 2016, I met Carla Bertolucci, who cultivated the ancient grain in Italy. Einkorn wheat is nature's original wheat from over 5000 years ago. It is organic, glyphosate free, and never hybridized. From an internal inquiry, I determined that this remedy would have a message for humanity. To these ends, I oversaw a homeopathic proving to deduce it properties.

Einkorn has to do with fertility and mothers nurturing their babies. Demeter, the goddess of fertility, is seen wearing Einkorn shafts in her hair. Einkorn has to do with humans connecting to animals and nature, and to the soothing words of the Great Mother Earth that houses us:

> **Survival of the human race is under the jurisdiction and influence of child bearing women. It is up to women to change the trajectory of current day economics, politics, and agricultural practices to ensure survival of the human race.**

The message of Einkorn is to release our fear and undo the centuries of power structures that perpetuate male over female dominance, Man over earth dominance, war, famine, and the economic prisons we hold in our minds. Einkorn wants us to return to the paradise we once had here on earth when we lived in accordance to nature's laws.

By eating Einkorn, it normalizes digestive and biliary functions, that release fear of inadequacy and feelings of lack and want (as dysfunction in these organs are associated with those feelings). Einkorn facilitates discernment by way of stripping away thousands of years of control, deprecation, fear, and suppression of our true nature by patriarchal power structures. By eating cultured Einkorn, as in sourdough products, it not only facilities healthy bile creation and feelings of wellbeing, it also introduces healthy lacto-fermenting bacteria into the intestines thus increasing tryptophan and phenylalanine necessary for healthy neurotransmitter function.

The resultant increased serotonin gives an expanded sense of joy and belonging. Over time, from eating Einkorn, you will feel incredibly satiated, not only physically but mentally and emotionally. By taking the remedy ***Triticum monococcum***, the centuries of wrong thinking and cultural myths that impress upon us naturally dissolve. The fear and lies will be forgotten and the truth we will remain. Einkorn empowers you to live, and frees your spirit to utilize your mind and body for the higher purposes of this existence.

To learn more about Einkorn view the movie on YouTube: https://www.youtube.com/watch?v=T7FjJCmufhQ.

Paradise Lost and Found

A homeopathic proving of Triticum monococcum - Einkorn wheat

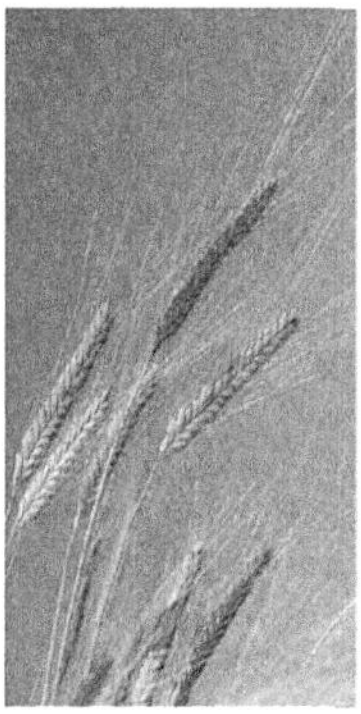

Experience the consciousness of Nature's original wheat: Einkorn (Triticum monococcum). Einkorn was the first food of the agrarian age. Now, when humanity is on the brink of its own extinction, through the pollution of this world and ourselves, the message of Einkorn is loud and clear: "We must live in accordance to Nature's Laws if we are to survive."

Kate Birch, RSHom(NA), is a book author, lecturer and an international expert in infectious disease, homeoprophylaxis and treating vaccine injury. She has applied the Genus Epidemicus model of homeopathic philosophy in search of a remedy that will help humanity come to its senses about who we really are. The food we eat determines who we will become.

View here: **https://youtu.be/T7FjJCmufhQ**

Vaccinefree.wordpress.com

---

cxl Sophie Ochmann, Max Roser. Polio. November 2017. Our World in Data. https://ourworldindata.org/polio.

11. Nutritional Support for the Detox Protocol

While the directions that follow may look like it is easy to detoxify your system from glyphosate, and one may question why we might need to change the global use of this poison, this protocol will not protect you from future exposure nor will it completely address the chronicity of many the health conditions created. Vigilance to your diet, your spending dollars, and political action is what will change this trajectory.

Here we begin to create order!

Basic Detox Steps:

A. Clean up food sources and exposure incidence: **Table One: Avoid These Foods**.
B. Consider **Fast and Colon Cleanse** to facilitate healthy kidney and liver function.
C. **Meal planning**: To repair the intestinal lining and immune system function with functional nutrition.
D. Add nutritional detoxification plan: **Table Two: Foods to Nourish**.
E. Add mechanical detoxification plan: **Table Three: Mechanical Support**.
F. Add homeopathic treatment and **Glyphosate Clearing Protocol**.
G. Maintain vigilance towards future exposure to glyphosate.

A. **Clean your Cupboards**: Before embarking on any kind of cleanse one must examine all foods that are being consumed. ALL commercial grade foods have some level of contamination. ALL GMO foods have been sprayed with glyphosate. Many household products contain glyphosate and/or the detergents that increase cell permeability and resultant toxicity. Use vinegar, salt, or baking soda for cleaning. The use of detergents and fragrances will maintain a leaky cell permeability which encourages increased uptake of glyphosate into your cells: remove them from your home and lifestyle.

Do not consume these foods: remove from diet and house immediately. This food is dead and should not be consumed out of principle (nature manipulated to satisfy addictions, economic and political agendas: e.g. sugar addictions; embargo on importation of sugar from Cuba).	
NO GMO foods or non-organic foods. No wheat or oats. **No** non-organic lentils, peas, soybeans, corn, flax, rye, triticale, buckwheat, millet, canola, sugar beets, grapes, potatoes, or sunflower seeds. Plants producing oils may also be treated pre-harvest with glyphosate.	GMO products are made so they can withstand glyphosate; this means these foods are made to be resistant to glyphosate so that it does not kill the plant. Glyphosate is used to desiccate a wide range of other crops.
NO grains except organic wild rice or Einkorn wheat.	No grains, except wild rice and organically grown Einkorn wheat, as they have been hybridized and/or genetically modified. Einkorn is the original wheat that has never been hybridized or genetically modified.
NO refined sugar. Sugar cane is highly sprayed.	This feeds the glyphosate driven *Candida* populations taking over your body.
NO high-fructose corn syrup, artificial sweeteners, or colorants.	High-fructose corn syrup is processed from glyphosate sprayed corn. Aspartame is a neurotoxin driving excessive dopamine. Artificial colorants act as neurotoxins as well.
NO tobacco	Heavily sprayed and bad for you.

NO commercial milk, animal products, or eggs.	Animal sources fed with GM are contaminated with glyph
NO Gelatin (Jell-O). Unless it is from organic and 100% grass-fed animal sources.	This is made from animal col on glyphosate contaminated g s.
NO processed foods or fast foods.	Most likely GMO, devoid of any enzymes, and contaminated with glyphosate and trans-fats.
NO antibiotics.	Kills the biome. Commensal bacteria are necessary for all digestive and regulatory processes in the body. They help in the creation of neurotransmitters and DNA or RNA regulation. Antibiotics promote the excessive growth of candida, antibiotic resistant bacteria, and iron deficiency. Glyphosate is also an antibiotic.
NO vaccines.	Incubated on gelatin (collagen) and fed bovine casein from cows fed GMO grains contaminated with glyphosate. Vaccines propel glyphosate driven inflammation. Vaccines import viral strains that under the influence of glyphosate may remain active.
No California wines. Other wines from around the world may be equally contaminated.	All grape crops are heavily sprayed. If we all stop drinking these wines, we can change the economy of California. Glyphosate causes paralyzing headaches and sleepiness.
No MSG.	Monosodium glutamate: used as a flavor enhancer increases glutamate toxicity.

B. **Fast and Colon Cleanse**: If you have never done any kind of detoxication process it is recommended that you do a full 10-day cleanse before embarking on a detox specifically trying to eliminate glyphosate. This 10-day program will clear years of built-up stool in the intestines so your body will more readily be able to detox glyphosate from your cells and liver. See 18. **Fast and Colon Cleanse**. To clear glyphosate, all eliminatory organs need to be working well. Fasting also helps reduce the toxic load on the body and increase nicotinamide adenine dinucleotide (NAD) levels which facilitates all autoregulatory processes and detoxing pathways in the body.

C. **Meal Planning**: If you eat a regular organic whole food diet, there is not much more you would need to add or eliminate to your regime. Those who are used to consuming fast food, a lot of wheat, and GMO food will have to convert your diet. This may take several weeks to adjust. Wait until this transition is complete before starting detoxification.

D. Follow the guidelines listed on **Table Two** for nutritional support of glyphosate detoxification. Plan to eat 2-3 meals a day. This is not a hard and fast schedule. Most supplements can be purchased online, through health care practitioners, and/or health food stores. The supplements listed in **Table Two** can all be consumed at the same time, 2-3 times a day, with meals, and hydration. On the days you take homeopathic ***Glyphosate*** in accordance to the **Glyphosate Clearing Protocol** be sure to take the psyllium husks, charcoal, and bentonite clay, for mechanical support to your colon and body.

Simple Dietary Guidelines:

- **Eat organic** (note many organic foods may be contaminated).
- **Eat Local. Grow** your own food.
- Eat 100% organic **Grass-fed** or 100% **Free-Range** animal products.
- **Become a farmer** to repair the soil from toxicity and reintroduce the much-needed soil biome for sustainable agriculture (which may take five to ten years).

The Weston A. Price Nourishing Traditions diet is ideal for the detox process.[cxli] If too much damage to the intestinal lining has occurred from excessive antibiotics or other demonstrations of leaky gut syndrome, the GAPS diet, primarily based on bone broth, may be needed to repair the damage prior to embarking on a glyphosate cleanse. See ***Polio*** nosode to help down regulate zonulin and close tight junctions. Ensure the animal sources for bone broth are 100% organic grass-fed. Continuation with the GAPS diet after the detox process will secure maintenance of health.

The **Glyphosate Clearing Protocol** is to be done while you are eating an all organic grain free diet (with the addition of Einkorn wheat or wild rice). If you are not yet organic or grain free, it takes several weeks to convert your pantry before embarking on the supplementation and detox phase of the **Glyphosate Clearing Protocol**.

Remember, you are what you eat. If you eat a toxin you will become toxic. The state of mind of that toxin will affect your state of mind. Pesticides and herbicides are against life. Life is all interconnected. The homicidal and suicidal inclinations in this society reflect the outward manifestation of the toxins affecting us. When we clean up our food our spirit will be free. If you are feeling suicidal, please be sure to reach out to a practitioner or suicide hotline.

Plan to spend at least 8-10 weeks adhering to this nutritional support along with mechanical detox, homeopathic treatment, and the **Glyphosate Clearing Protocol**.

E. **Mechanical Support**: this kind of support augments the nutritional detoxification process to release glyphosate from the liver and collagen stores in the body: See **Table Three**.
F. **Homeopathic Support**.
G. **Glyphosate Clearing Protocol.**

---

cxli Fallon, Sally. Nourishing Traditions. New Trends Publishing, Inc.; 2nd Revised edition (2001).

and scheduling of supplementation and nutrition, expounded upon below, is to be taken during the homeopathic **Glyphosate Clearing Protocol**. Adjust to needs. These foods/supplements are listed in order of priority.

It may be necessary to do the **Fast and Colon Cleanse** prior to beginning to detox glyphosate to ensure elimination pathways are open. A glyphosate detox is not the same as the **Fast and Colon Cleanse.** In this detox we want to eat all the good foods to rebuild the body and assist detoxification with the additional procedures and supplements.

Foods and Supplements	Why	Suggested Dosage
	Biome and Enzymes	
Fermented foods such as kombucha, yogurt, kefir, and sauerkraut. Sourdough Einkorn wheat. Raw milk, probiotics. Mix up sources. Rhubarb.	To replace and maintain the biome that has been destroyed by glyphosate. Bacteria are necessary for many digestive functions, the production of enzymes, fatty acids, neurotransmitters, and regulation of all hormones. Also, to combat the overgrowth of *Candida*. Raw milk is full of natural bacteria and enzymes. Probiotics with inulin or lactoferrin (both prebiotics) helps to repopulate the intestines. Rhubarb maintains high pH regulating the intestinal biome. Inulin is a soluble fiber found in many plants which helps to maintain healthy bacterial balance. These bacteria then convert inulin to short-chain fatty acids.	Daily: multiple times.

Foods and Supplements	Why	Dosage
Biome and Enzymes		
Digestive enzymes. Miso, papaya, fermented foods, raw milk, raw foods and juices.	To replace the digestive enzymes that have been inactivated by glyphosate, or that are not being created by the crippled DNA/RNA coded protein sequences and deficient bacterial populations. To help with the digestion of all food.	3 capsules- 3 times a day with meals. Add to diet regularly.
Soil enzymes and bacteria.	Soil organisms help to restore intestinal lining by down regulating zonulin and repairing the tight junctions. They produce fulvic acid and humic acid that binds to glyphosate then metabolizes it so it can be released from the system.	As per re-commended dosing.
Raw apple cider vinegar.	Vinegar is a blood astringent and cellular detoxifier. It is rich in enzymes and acetic acid. Apple cider vinegar microbes, *acetobacter*, metabolize glyphosate. Acetobacter is a genus of bacteria that reduces lactic acid by oxidizing lactate and acetate into carbon dioxide and water. Raw apple cider vinegar helps the liver release bile acids to digest fats, clean the blood, and normalize pH. It also helps with weight loss. Too much can lead to excessive weight loss. Apple cider vinegar helps to increase iron, and reduce excess adenosine, and deactivate its receptor sites.	At least 1 tsp /day. No more than 1 Tbsp per day.

Foods and Supplements	Why	Dosage
Biome and Enzymes		
Raw apple cider or juice.	High in pectin and malic acid to clean the liver, break up gallstones and kidney stones and other detox pathways in the liver. Helps in the formation of bile acids.	4 oz./day, mix with collagen.
L- glutamine.	Helps convert glutamate to GABA. Works to calm the system.	Daily.
SAMe	S-adenosylmethionine: synthesized from adenosine triphosphate (ATP) and methionine by methionine adenosyl transferase. Methionine is an essential amino acid which serves as the substrate for other amino acids like glutathione. It serves as a regulator in a variety of processes including DNA and RNA transcription, the methylation to glutathione, immune response, amino acid metabolism, the folate pathway, transsulfuration, and more. Normally it is found in whole grains and dairy and is synthesized in the liver or by the enterobacteria *(E. coli)*. Supplementation comes from the bacteria. SAMe is essential for the creation of histamine-N-methyltransferase which serves to break down histamine (more specifically excess histamine in the brain) thus reducing cerebral inflammation.	One tablet daily.

Foods and Supplements	Why	Dosage
Biome and Enzymes		
Cobalamin (B12) and Folate (B9) supplementati on if *Bifidobacteria* deficient.	Healthy brain development, neurulation, fetal viability, and development and regulation of hormones and neurotransmitters. Necessary for the methylation of glutathione needed for detoxification. Deficiencies are implicit to MTHFR gene mutations.	As directed.
5-HTP.	To replace missing tryptophan due to dysbiosis. Necessary precursor to serotonin formation and its 5-HT receptors.	1-5 a day.
Glycine, Collagen, and Bone Broth		
Collagen: from all organic grass-fed beef or organically grain-fed chicken, seaweed, and fish sources. No farm-raised fish.	Absolutely necessary to repair the weakened collagen in the body and to replace glyphosate with glycine. By doing this switch routine on a daily basis the system will be flooded with glycine and will naturally release the glyphosate competitor. Collagen sources also include varying levels of the non-essential amino acids: alanine, arginine, aspartic acid, glutamic acid, hydroxylysine, proline, serine, and tyrosine. And the essential amino acids: histidine, isoleucine, leucine, lysine, methionine, phenylalanine, threonine, and valine.	1 scoop (2 tbsp) 2-4 times a day. Mix with warm water to dissolve, add juice for flavor.
Foods high in glycine.	Plant-based sources include beans; vegetables like spinach, kale, cauliflower, cabbage, and pumpkin; plus, fruits like banana and kiwi.	Daily: can be consumed with all that is listed here.

	Other than bone broth, glycine can also be found in complete sources of proteins including meat, seafood, dairy products, poultry, eggs, and fish.	
Foods and Supplements	Why	Dosage
Glycine, Collagen, and Bone Broth		
Bone broth/ soups. Seaweed. Learn more about GAPS diet for full explanation.	High in Glycine and L-glutamine. Bone broth is necessary to repair the gut lining that has been destroyed by glyphosate. Glycine is necessary to build collagen in body. L-glutamine is necessary to normalize T1/T2 responses in the immune system, it facilitates detoxification processes, and balances glutamate and GABA ratios in the brain. Use lightly cooked stocks (30-60 min) if the intestinal lining is damaged and your system over produces histamine.	Daily: or several times per week.
Antioxidants, Blood Purification, Chelators		
Fat-soluble vitamin C: Ascorbyl palmitate.	Acts as an antioxidant to work with fats and oils to penetrate the cell membranes and enter the cells; to bind to and remove cell-bound glyphosate and free radicals. Vitamin C increases diamine oxidase (DAO) which oxidizes excess histamine This is especially needed during the **Glyphosate Clearing Protocol** but can be started along with digestive enzymes and other nutritional products prior. Vitamin C is necessary for a number of other enzymatic reactions such as conversion of folic	2-6 capsules (1000mg-4000mg) daily. Divide doses hourly: e.g. 2 capsules per hour.

	acid to folate (B9) and the functionality of the iron dependent enzyme aromatase needed for androgen conversion and iron assimilation.	
Foods and Supplements	Why	Dosage
Antioxidants, Blood Purification, Chelators		
Citrus: lemons, limes, grapefruit, oranges. All organic.	High in Vitamin C, citrate, potassium, calcium, phosphorus, magnesium, copper, thiamine (B1), riboflavin (B2), niacin (B3), pantothenic acid (B5), pyridoxine (B6), folate (B9), and a variety of phytochemicals and flavonoids. Citrus helps to prevent heart disease and kidney stones. Helps in the production of bile thus lowering cholesterol, facilities healthy cellular hydration, helps to absorb iron and other essential nutrients. Helps in the production of collagen and strengthens bones. Lemons especially help in the alkalization of the body (increases pH). High in inositol that facilitates the binding of neurotransmitters and hormones to their receptor sites. Citrus fruits can act as agonists to the muscarinic acetylcholine receptors (mAChRs).	Daily: fresh squeezed.
Pomegranate juice.	A blood astringent. Cleans the blood. Adds iron and vitamin C	4-6 oz./ day.
Turmeric, ginger and galangal root	Turmeric, high in curcumin helps to reduce systemwide inflammation. Curcumin works on local inflammation but also regulates the	Daily: use as tea, in your cooking, fresh juice

	genetic control of the immune system. Curcumin is an antioxidant, helps to increase the number and functionality of brain cells, reduces heart disease by cleaning the blood (astringent), reduce the number of and growth of cancer cells, and boosts levels of serotonin and dopamine. Ginger, high in gingerol, reduces inflammation because of its antioxidant properties It helps to reduce heart disease and high blood sugar (hyperglycemia), lowers cholesterol and helps the immune system work with co-infections and cancer. Galangal improves virility of sperm, increases blood circulation, and acts as an antioxidant, anti-cancer, antibacterial and anti-inflammatory agent.	
Antioxidants, Blood Purification, Chelators		
Hibiscus, rosehips, raspberry leaf tea, cranberry, or sarsaparilla.	All to increase the antioxidant vitamin C and help reduce excess adenosine levels by supplementing ADA. All act as antioxidants, blood astringents, and urinary tonifiers. Cranberry helps to increase adenosine triphosphate (ATP) levels and protect the kidneys. Sarsaparilla helps to protect the kidneys from heavy metal damage.	Daily: multiple sources.
Green onions and garlic.*	High in selenium and sulfur to help with metabolic and immune processes. *Caution for those with sulfur metabolism issues (MTHFR gene mutations).	Daily: often.

Foods and Supplements	Why	Dosage
Antioxidants, Blood Purification, Chelators		
Glutathione.	Supplementing glutathione levels reduces oxidative stress. This is needed in combination with B12 and folate (B9) in those with MTHFR gene mutations.	Daily.
Magnesium citrate.	To move bowels which eliminates the glyphosate being dumped into the intestines during detox. Magnesium citrate is an antioxidant that also binds oxalates and heavy metals, calms the nervous system, and reduces glutamate levels in the brain by facilitating glutamine synthetase(GS).	1-2 tsp/ day.
Sea salt.	For trace minerals and iodine. Necessary for T4 to T3 conversion and for healthy thyroid function. Helps to convert bile acids to bile salts and build appetite. Sea salt enemas, or overnight cleanse, will rinse colon of built up toxic residue from harbored old stool. For overnight cleanse take in solution, one gallon per 1/2 cup of salt to be drunk in 6 hours after midnight.	To taste. Take extra during saunas. Consider overnight salt water cleanse.
Herbal liver detox and support.	Celandine, dandelion, burdock root, milk thistle, aloe vera, barberry, and bitters. Parsley, thyme, and basil have micronutrients to help with sulfate transport. For more info: *Homeopathic Therapeutics of the Liver and Biliary Ducts ~ The Amazing Liver: Interfacing Nature with Spirit.* By Kate Birch.	

Foods and Supplements	Why	Dosage
Basic Nutrition		
Oils and Fats: animal fat, coconut oil, fish oil. Avocados.	Necessary for insulating the brain and other vital organs from glyphosate toxicity. Necessary to repair cell membranes that have been degraded by glyphosate and detergents and to ensure they are receptive to the fat-soluble vitamin C. These are also necessary to make 'good' cholesterol.	Daily: multiple servings.
Super blue-green algae, micro algae, wheat grass, spirulina, chlorella, and super greens.	Super blue-green algae is high in manganese, amino acids and other trace minerals. May be the best super food on the market. Manganese helps with the uptake and functionality of iron. Blue-green algae contains varying levels of the non-essential amino acids: alanine, arginine, aspartic acid, glutamic acid, hydroxylysine, proline, serine, and tyrosine, and the essential amino acids: histidine, isoleucine, leucine, lysine, methionine, phenylalanine, threonine, and valine. Other algae sources may not contain all these nutrients.	Daily: 2-3 capsules.
Dehydrated beef liver extract.* *This food is high in purines. If you have tendency	Organ meats nourish the body deeply. The liver is high in iron, replacing deficiencies created by glyphosate and a high *Candida* load. High yeast leads to anemia. High yeast is also an indication of mercury or heavy metal toxicity and hyper-acidic body. Iron is necessary for all heme-dependent	1 tbsp per day mixed with apple or pineapple juice.

towards gout use sparingly or not at all.	CYP protein enzyme creation and thyroid function. *Pesticides and herbicides are heavily used in Argentina (main sources for this product. Contamination with glyphosate is likely. Seek out alternative sources	
Foods and Supplements	Why	Dosage
Basic Nutrition		
Oysters and mollusks.	Oysters are a super food. High in protein, vitamins, and omega 3s. Vitamins A, C, D, E, K and B vitamins: thiamine (B1), riboflavin (B2), niacin (B3), pantothenic acid (B5), pyridoxine (B6), biotin (B7), folate (B9), and cobalamin (B12). High in choline (essential for acetylcholine) and betaine (prevents the buildup of homocysteine). High in calcium, iron, magnesium, phosphorus, sodium, zinc, copper, manganese, selenium and fluorine. Choline, calcium, and zinc together facilitate many physiological processes related to the nicotinic acetylcholine receptor sites (nAChRs).	Often: weekly, 2-5 per serving.
Digestive fiber: organic lentils, beans.	Necessary to keep bowels regular and to cleanout old debris in colon.	1 -3 servings per day.
Eggs.	High in nutrients, sulfur, and cholesterol needed to help detox glyphosate.	Often.

Foods and Supplements	Why	Dosage
Basic Nutrition		
Minerals: zinc, sulfur, selenium, iron, iodine, molybdenum, manganese, cobalt.	To improve enzymatic activity, vitamin formation, ligand bound GPCR site function, nutritional metabolism, absorption, and functional implications of each of these minerals. All this is to help with healthy methylation cycles and thyroid function which may be interfered with by glyphosate's disruption of the enzymatic processes' dependent on these nutrients.	As per recommended daily amounts.
Stinging nettles: fresh or dried in tea.	High in vitamins A and C, calcium, iron, amino acids, and the fatty acids: oleic, linoleic, palmitic and omega-3. High in chlorophyll (manganese), phosphate, calcium, potassium, sodium and other minerals. Includes the essential amino acids: threonine, valine, isoleucine, leucine, phenylalanine, lysine, histidine, and methionine.	2-3 cups a day. Boil water, add nettles, steep all day, strain, drink at room temp.
Excess clean and clear water: Fiji water or Volvic water.	To keep the body hydrated and pH balanced to facilitate detox; water high in silicates helps immune system and detox pathways.	At least 1 quart/ day.

Foods and Supplements	Why	Dosage
Not to be consumed with supplements		
Mechanical Binding Agents		
Activated charcoal and bentonite clay.	To absorb the glyphosate dumped in the intestines and other old compacted stool debris. Do not consume at the same time as food or supplements as those will be absorbed and eliminated with these binders. Best time for this is last thing before bed.	Charcoal: 4-8 capsules /day. Clay: 1-2 tsp /day. Drink with lots of water.
Psyllium husks.	Adds fiber and helps to bind with debris in the intestines and colon. Can be consumed with bentonite clay and charcoal	Consume with plenty of water.

Enemas: coffee enema, lemon rinse, sea salt rinse, probiotic implant enema, at least once a week. More often at the beginning of the cleanse.	Necessary if your bowels are blocked and stopped up. Also, as you detox glyphosate it is kind of like glue and will get sticky in the intestines. Coffee enemas can pull old stool out. Salt rinses change osmotic potential across the intestinal lining allowing for detox. Lemon rinse will reset pH. Probiotic implant puts healthy bacteria in the lower intestines. Do it in this order: clean, reset pH, then re-establish biome. 1-4 times during protocol, especially in the beginning to make sure intestines are clean and eliminating all waste. See 18. **Fast and Colon Cleanse** for more info on how to do an enema.
Sauna, hot tub, hot bath, or infrared sauna: daily, weekly, often.	Heat is required for releasing and relaxing the collagen fibers so glyphosate can be released. Be sure to be well hydrated and salted prior to sauna. Consume activated charcoal and bentonite clay in the hours before and after sauna to bind with the liberated glyphosate. Skin may break out in ulcers during this process. Infrared light creates heat and light to help this process.
Epson salts in the bath.	Magnesium sulphate in the bath helps to provide sulfur transdermally to facilitate methylation pathways for detoxification.
Massage or Rolfing: several times throughout the detox protocol.	Massage for cellular health and detox. Rolfing, which is specific for working on the fascia (collagen) where glyphosate gets stored in the body. This activates immune system cells in the fascia to engage them in the immunological process of triggering macrophages to remove damaged tissue and cells.
Skin rubbing while bathing.	To release glyphosate from the superficial cellular levels.

Massage of viscera of the intestines.	The viscera of the intestinal system and omentum of the stomach will be loaded with glyphosate as this is the first line of exposure. The surrounding fascia of the intestines and particularly surrounding the ileocecal valve is where the highest concentration is held. When this area of the body is impacted by glyphosate it causes a contraction in the fascia of the spine leading to spinal contortion. This can extend up to the base of the skull causing headaches and pain along the spine. During the detox, and subsequently, daily massage of the ileocecal valve and intestinal viscera is necessary to manipulate the glyphosate out. Through this manipulation it will be pulled into the circulatory system to the liver or directly into the intestines. It can also filter through the kidneys to be eliminated in the urine as it is water soluble.
Yoga: weekly, multiple times.	Increased cellular oxygenation. Cellular oxygenation raises pH and reduces lactic acid. Yoga stretches fascia to release glyphosate so it is ready to be picked up by the white blood cells/lymphatic system directly to the large intestine or to be detoxed through the liver and then large intestines. Note: in the beginning you will feel more toxic after yoga unless you have the other detox pathways open. Be sure to do some cleansing activity and hydrate before and after yoga. Be sure to add collagen before yoga to take up the glycine into your fascia during your practice. The more you stretch the fascia, the more the glycine will be absorbed, and glyphosate will be released. Yoga is also about realizing your oneness with GOD. Yoga is about self-realization which is GOD-realization.

Meditation.	To build self-awareness and presence of being that connects you to all. To facilitate the transformation of humans from destroying themselves to living in harmony with their pure essence and the natural world that hosts their consciousness. To set the stage for the activation of your free will.
Action.	Now that you know all this, plan what you can do to be in service to fix this problem not only in yourself, but for your children and fellow man. Your survival is dependent upon your actions.

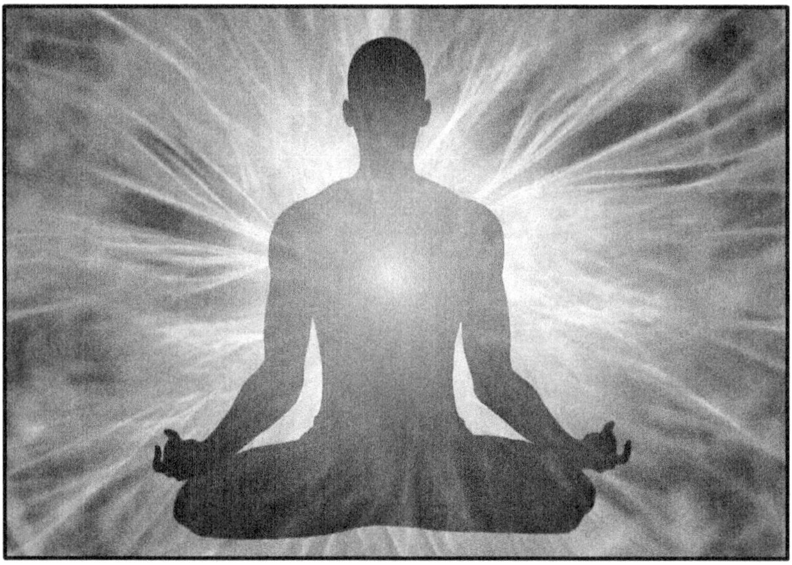

12. Final Notes and Review

1. Core supplementation is:
    a. Fat-soluble vitamin C: 1000 mg per day.
    b. Digestive enzymes: 3 capsules three times a day.
    c. Probiotics: 2 capsule 3 times a day.
    d. Collagen powder: one scoop twice a day.
2. You need to eat all organic foods. Especially meat, dairy, and poultry. Make sure they are not grain fed. 100% grass-fed food sources only. You also need to eat a high fat diet and implement an ocean sourced-, chicken-, or beef-based collagen. No GMO or pesticide spayed foods ever.

1. No use of perfumes, detergents, or other toxins as glyphosate is often combined with these detergents and other ingredients that heighten its absorbability into the cells of plants that are sprayed. These also increase the permeability of your cells. Personal use of fragrances and detergent products make the removal of glyphosate that much harder. Clean your house and cupboards of all perfumes.
2. Vaccines are made on growth mediums such as gelatin (animal-based collagen) which are fed GMO "Roundup-Ready" grain feed and therefore have glyphosate in them. Also, they use non-organic, GMO-fed, bovine and porcine blood serums as nutrient bases which contain glyphosate. Never vaccinate. There are other options such as homeoprophylaxis.
3. We need a diet rich in fermented foods, healthy bacteria, and digestive enzymes to begin the process of repairing the intestinal lining and preparing to eliminate glyphosate.
4. To release the improperly placed glyphosate from protein chains we need to consume multiple digestive enzymes to enable the cleavage of disulphide bonds and use homeopathic remedies to help in this process (based on symptom presentation). See 15. **Homeopathic Remedies to Repair Glyphosate Damage**.
5. To open the secondary, tertiary, and quaternary (sulfur) bonds of proteins we first need heat such as infrared, hot baths, or saunas. Epson salts (magnesium sulphate) facilitate cellular detoxification and the opening of quaternary bonds. Your skin may break out in small ulcers as you release glyphosate.

6. Then we need digestive enzymes to access the glyphosate which has been inserted in the primary amino acid chains.
7. We also need to supplement with collagen to make the normal amino acid glycine more readily available to replace the newly released glyphosate.
8. Due to glyphosate induced dysbiosis, to get the newly ingested collagen (glycine) into the blood stream and to rebuild your fascia, you need mega doses of probiotics and enzymes in your digestive track.
9. As glyphosate is also held inside cells, we need to eat a high fat diet and take fat-soluble vitamin C (Ascorbyl Palmitate) to open the phospholipid membrane, so glyphosate can easily be released. Most glyphosate used commercially is also attached to detergents which make cells more permeable: as glyphosate is water soluble normally it would not enter cells unless these detergents are added to get past the phospholipid membrane. These detergents are more easily processed out of the body leaving the glyphosate trapped in the cells. Fat-soluble vitamin C is an antioxidant and acts as a reverse detergent, binding to and pulling out toxins for elimination. Our immune system helps to identify what is toxic. Our DNA is coded towards health, not disease. It will recognize disease producing substances, and respond accordingly, if unencumbered. DNA can repair itself and will edit glyphosate out if given the correct information. Vitamin C is also to help increase diamine oxidase (DAO) which oxidizes excess histamine thereby lowering inflammation.
10. The glycine consumed in healthy foods will normally enter cells through the ion channels in the cell membranes. By saturating the system with glycine, the hope is it takes the place of glyphosate in all subsequent protein synthesis.
11. Green onions are high in sulfur and selenium needed for absorbing glycine and methylation pathways. Cobalamin (B12) and folate (B9) may also be needed, especially with MTHFR gene mutations. Remember you can become selenium deficient in glyphosate toxicity, so supplementation may be necessary. Digestive enzymes are primary to the uptake of selenium.
12. Once the released glyphosate is in the blood, it needs to be escorted to the liver for detoxification with the fat-soluble vitamin

C (Ascorbyl Palmitate). As an antioxidant, it binds to glyphosate. There it will be processed by the liver and eliminated via bile acids to the large intestine where it will destroy the biome once again.

13. Mega doses of probiotics are still needed in the upper and lower intestines so the digestive process can continue to do the work till the glyphosate is escorted out. Charcoal and bentonite clay are helpful to bind with the glue-like glyphosate discharge. Plant fiber (lentils and beans) and pectin are also helpful to keep the stools loose. Check that your lentils are organic and not grown in Canada as they are heavily sprayed with glyphosate there. Even if they are organic there may be drift contamination. Otherwise these are the best forms of fiber. Did I mention activated charcoal is needed here?
14. Glyphosate can be excreted through the kidneys and will cause some damage. Improperly metabolized purines lead to excess uric acid which also can damage the kidneys. This manifests in the skin and joints: gout, urticaria and/or nephritis for example. Additionally, with kidney damage, phosphates cannot be excreted and will pull calcium from the bones to reconcile this, making the bones weak and increasing the tendency to kidney stone formation. Be sure to supplement with nutrients that support healthy kidney function like cranberry.
15. Note that glyphosate is a metal chelator (essential metal nutrients and heavy metals). As it passes out of the kidneys it will take the metals with it, including iron and other metals necessary for specific enzymes to function. Sarsaparilla tincture will help to limit damage to the kidneys from chelated heavy metals.
16. Herbal support for the liver: celandine, dandelion root, burdock root, milk thistle, and bitters. If constipated, use aloe vera liquid in small doses or for a short period of time only or magnesium citrate to move the bowels. Remember the more glyphosate you release from the system the more temporarily disrupted your digestive system will become. Your tongue will taste like soap or may burn as the glyphosate is being freed.
17. Raw milk is a cholagogue (stimulates bile release) as are the herbs above. Einkorn wheat is also an effective cholagogue. Drinkable yogurt supplies the probiotics and pulls bile from the liver.

18. Your skin may break out in the process. Suicidal thoughts may come and go. Neurotransmitters will be affected. Stay clear.

    Pray and do yoga. The suicidal thoughts come not only from the effect on neurotransmitter deficit but also because this is the psychology of a poison that is killing humanity. Glyphosate is a medium of genocide. If you feel you are wanting to kill yourself, don't believe it. It is the poison talking. Seek professional help as needed.
19. Study your mind and the thoughts you perseverate on surrounding your own self-deprecation. Once you are aware you can let them go.

14. Introduction to Homeopathic Support

While the individual may look to this section to find a homeopathic remedy or two to treat themselves in their glyphosate detox process, the ultimate cleanse is to be free of the sickness in humanity that has led us to the point of poisoning our own food supply.

Correspondingly, as you study the information presented, imagine looking through an adjustable lens. One that can zoom in and out according to your scope and point of view. We could focus our treatment by zooming into a specific biological reaction in a specific organ system, back up to see the individual as a collection of organ systems and functions, or back up further to examine the nature of Man and how our dictates have led us here.

If we expand our perspective to contemplate living in the material world, incarnation, your soul's purpose, and healing of the collective ills at the root of this problem we might affect some change. This would be the larger perspective. Simultaneously, as specific remedies are discussed with respect to a certain set of symptoms, or for a specific condition, this does not minimalize the need of the reader to know or understand the larger totality of symptomatology attributed to that remedy. Thus, my commentary, limited or extensive, is not a direct reflection of the healing potential of any one remedy over another to

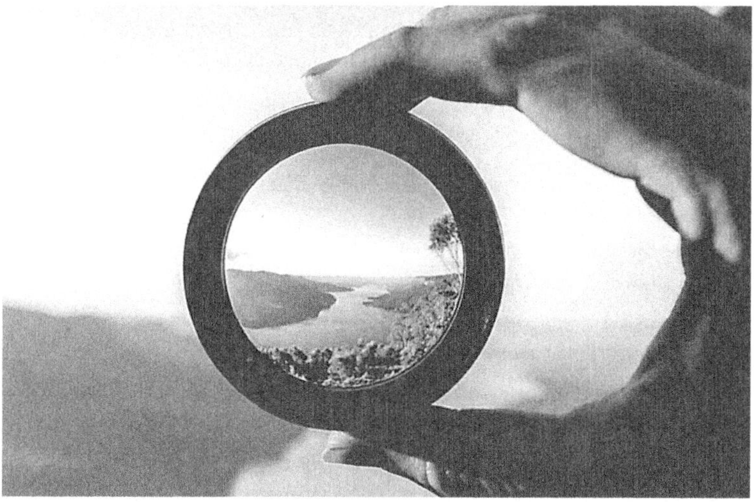

address any one aspect of a therapeutic focal point. One of my best teachers says we must prescribe for the largest meaningful

totality in that individual. If our prescriptions are spot on for the individual, we may in turn affect the larger totality in humanity. Collectively then, we can work towards realigning ourselves with the greater cosmic order.

Consequently, as I have researched, written, and contemplated this subject matter, I have examined my own survivability, questioned the potential of homeopathy, and that of nature, to resolve this issue. My small human-animal self has many doubts, my faith in humanity is next to nil. Yet my confidence in the healing vital force of nature and the ability of the earth to rebalance does not faulter. The question of whether humans will survive the earth's resolution to this problem is a different matter. Whether homeopathy alone can change the trajectory is also a question. It is this question that has led me to look deeper: in so doing, I am marveled at the genius of nature and how plant, mineral, and animal substances, when in potency, have the potential to heal our ailments and bring us closer to life, truth, and divinity. Through this, my own confidence in the road towards becoming glyphosate free is growing.

In this section an in-depth review or proof of homeopathic philosophy and potency are not explained or discussed. I will assume that if the reader has made it this far in this essay you are either curious, have consulted with a practitioner, or already know how to use homeopathy. That said, for the homeopathic practitioner, there is a considerable leap in thought process of translating the language of the clinical conditions of glyphosate toxicity to that of the language of homeopathic Materia Medica. I have done my best to make these jumps for you when possible while discussing remedies and clinical conditions. Before prescribing any of the remedies mentioned please confirm your selection and symptom presentation with more complete Materia Media volumes.

The basis of homeopathic understanding is that all living things are animated by a dynamic vital force. This Vital Force is connected to the unified field of existence (**Generating-Organizing-Delivering/ Destroying system**). Disease symptom expression in the human is also a part of that unified field and upon the planet are individual substances that mirror specific disease expressions. It follows that these substances are indicated to be the helpers that will return the system to balance. As we heal so does the planet.

Normally, homeopathic remedies are selected through symptom similarity between the subjective report to the pathogenesis of a remedy rather than diagnostic terms or laboratory tests. However, therapeutic remedy indications discussed here are grouped according to clinical conditions in order to maintain consistency in this narrative. Individuation in remedy selection must be made according to the homeopathicity of a symptom totality.

Detoxification of glyphosate requires mechanical, microbial, nutritional, herbal, and homeopathic interventions. Depending on which body system seems most affected, one or more of these approaches will produce the best results.

1. Glyphosate primarily needs to be physically removed from the body (mechanical and nutritional intervention).
2. To correct microbial balance, healthy microbes must be introduced.
3. Changes in functionality of system processes needs medicinal action (herbal and homeopathic intervention).
4. Homeopathic remedies are especially important to correct the energetic and functional disturbances resultant from glyphosate toxicity.

The purpose of homeopathic detoxification is to help the body differentiate what is not natural to the body and to facilitate freeing the system to release it. In so doing, our free will automatically come closer to the will of nature. Releasing the toxin is the natural outcome of using isopathic remedies (potentization preparations of the same substance that caused the problem). This is called Tautopathy. This process is not like chelation which mechanically binds to the toxin to be discharged. That is accomplished with herbal and nutritional support (charcoal, bentonite clay, etc.). Nor is it like using herbals to force biological responses in specific organs, pull bile, produce discharge, etc.

With the precept that, by design, the healthy functioning of the human animal is modulated by self-regulating and self-correcting mechanisms, by giving the potentized isopathic energetic information of the problem/issue, the body will naturally self-correct and voluntarily open the eliminatory pathways to remove the toxin. The time it takes, and the number of doses, is dependent on how severe the issue is to begin with. We can only hope that we can correct the much larger disaster that "Big Ag" has done to us and the earth. Time will tell.

There is no known research on homeopathic treatment of glyphosate toxicity. The information herein is based on my clinical experience and needs to be further evaluated in clinical practice. While homeopathy is a 200-year-old system of medicine, the manmade disease of glyphosate toxicity is new, it is not natural disease, and is difficult to treat. Additionally, you might get the impression from these writings that glyphosate is easy to clear from the body or to correct the imbalances it produces. It is not. It disarms all processes fundamental to life starting at how DNA and RNA functions. To fix that takes a miracle. Homeopathy is part of the puzzle.

The tautopathic (isopathic) remedies used in the detox process are not available over the counter, nor from most homeopathic pharmacies. You would need to work with a CEASE trained homeopathic practitioner to have access to them.

Homeopathic Treatment Approaches: It is up to the practitioner to be able to sort out the differences in philosophical approaches as they find and apply the appropriate remedies. Detoxification is a layering process, start with the most critical or foundational layer first. E.g. addressing gut biome and enzyme deficiency is primary, the asthma, gout, cancer, etc. is secondary. For the novice, this section is for you to understand what avenue your homeopath may use. While classical homeopathy asserts that there is only one disease at a time in an individual and while natural disease may express its dysfunction in multiple systems as one symptom totality, glyphosate toxicity is a manmade disease manifesting in multiple unrelated systems and may need a variety of remedies to fully address its' effects.

It is true that while glyphosate will affect the weakest links in that individual, thus exposing the chronic susceptibility, its toxic effects are unique to it and a tautopathic approach is necessary (e.g. ***Glyphosate*** or ***RoundUp*** remedy).

Points of View:

1. **Classical Homeopathy**: This is the use of a single homeopathic remedy (same disease) at a time to address constitutional health which is a result of natural disease processes of the individual in relation to the life they live.
2. **Clinical Homeopathy**: That which may include more than one remedy at a time, at differing potency levels, to support not only constitutional issues but also specific organs. This may include bowel nosodes, disease nosodes, cell salts, herbal preparations, etc. My understanding is glyphosate toxicity needs this approach.
   For Example:
   - Organ specific herbal tinctures in crude dose.
   - Functional system/discharge specific cell salts in X potency in the a.m.
   - Daily dose of constitutional remedy in 30C Monday to Friday in the p.m.
   - Bowel nosodes in 200C or 1M weekly.
   - Nosodes and/or sarcodes in 30C, 200C, or 1M, depending.
   - Consider addressing the biome with Bowel nosodes and remedies initially while the person is sorting out their diet and eliminatory system. Progress to deeper prescribing as you begin to understand the case more.
   - Intercurrent different remedies at paces and in potencies as needed. If using multiple remedies in sequential dosing, it is best to use varied potencies so each can work in its plane of frequency.
   - Commence with the **Glyphosate Clearing Protocol** after you have corrected the gut biome and ensured health eliminatory aspects of the liver and kidneys.

3. **Single Dose Verses Daily Dose**: In Kentian Homeopathy it is more common to give a single dose of a high potency remedy seldomly (some call this Classical Homeopathy). In toxicity cases, a lower potency repeated more often will effect greater cure because there is the maintaining cause of glyphosate in the system.
4. **Miasmatic Prescribing**: The use of miasmatic disease nosodes in addition to classical homeopathy or clinical homeopathy.
5. **Homeopathic Detoxing Protocols-Tautopathy**: This is the isopathic (same disease) use of the drug or chemical which has caused the damage in the first place. In this case it is the use of ***Glyphosate*** or ***RoundUp*** in ascending potencies. Toxicity issues are man-made diseases and the resolution of these conditions requires that these toxins, as operators in the system, must be removed by in-kind remedies in an ascending potency scale (30C, 200C, 1M, 10M). The concurrent pathogenesis must be treated at the same time as detoxification by remedies that match the symptom picture or support the organs afflicted by that toxicity.
6. **Vaccine Detox-CEASE Therapy**: While it is not in the scope of this book to discuss vaccine detox, it is important to mention as prior vaccines can set up a chronic inflammatory condition, or increase gut permeability by upregulation of zonulin. The co-morbidity of glyphosate toxicity and vaccine induced inflammation needs to be addressed by first doing a vaccine detox. Vaccine issues can also be addressed with tautopathy (remedies made from the vaccines given). All conditions induced by vaccines and the aluminum adjuvants in vaccines are compounded by glyphosate toxicity. Correspondingly, resolution of vaccine injury must be accompanied with the removal from the diet of all glyphosate sprayed products and the addition of associated homeopathic remedies to address the common areas of disruption. A vaccine detox must be embarked upon prior to homeopathic glyphosate detox to remove the infectious disease agents that are driving the inflammation. Remove all glyphosate riddled food (gluten, dairy, and non-organic foods) while doing the vaccine detox.
7. **Heavy Metal Detox**: The same is true here. Glyphosate toxicity compounds heavy metal toxicity, which also affects the biome by

driving up *Candida* populations. If so poisoned, aim to detox the metals first nutritionally and homeopathically then follow with glyphosate clearing. Reason being is that *Candida* overgrowth, which is common to heavy metal toxicity, is present to save the body from the metal toxicity. If you take the *Candida* away without addressing the metals, you may increase the damage to organs from the heavy metals. Heavy metal detoxification is not discussed in this presentation. That said, as glyphosate reduces the glutathione levels in the liver, glutathione is needed to eliminate heavy metals. You may need to revisit a heavy metal detox once you have completed your first round of the **Glyphosate Clearing Protocol**. Be sure to supplement with glutathione while doing a heavy metal detox.

Homeopathic Detox Process: Prior to embarking on the homeopathic **Glyphosate Clearing Protocol** we need to ensure the large intestine is mechanically eliminating properly before introducing homeopathic remedies that will support the process. The **Fast and Colon Cleanse** gives instructions on how to do this. The tables on nutritional and mechanical support cover how to support detox pathways.

Constitutional remedies will help those areas of the individual's health that have been disrupted by glyphosate and also the soil upon which this happened. After a few weeks of constitutional homeopathic support, followed by nutritional preparation and repair of the intestinal biome, we then add the **Glyphosate Clearing Protocol**. If the exposure is specifically Roundup or if you are extremely sensitive to smells, then a **Roundup Clearing Protocol** maybe needed. This would be accomplished in the same manner or done after the **Glyphosate Clearing Protocol**.

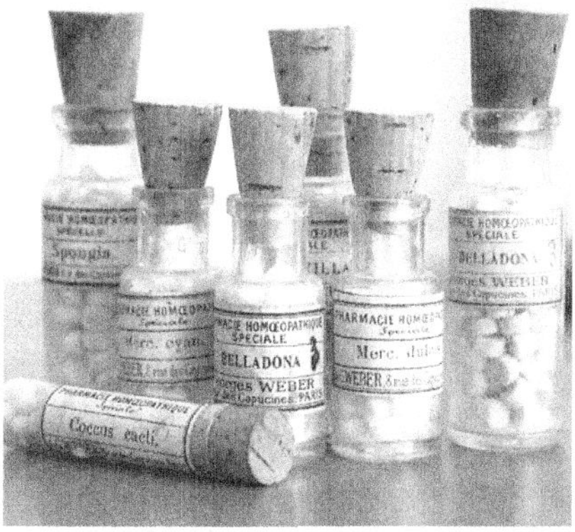

Case Taking: Take the initial case just as you would in regular practice. If you suspect glyphosate toxicity, hone your focus to which specific organ system or cellular function is the most affected. Three or more conditions in the following symptom collection would lead you to suspect probable glyphosate toxicity. Support the nutritional detox and **Glyphosate Clearing Protocol** with the most indicated constitutional remedies.

- Cannot digest wheat. Gluten intolerance, bloating from wheat. Says they can eat wheat in Europe.
- Systemic food intolerances.
- Headaches from wine or beer. Blinding headaches before menses. Right-sided headaches.
- Systemic inflammation. Gout.
- Lives in agricultural lands. Works as a baker or farmer.
- Sensitive to smells, perfumes, and detergents.
- Unexplained bronchospasm or asthma.
- Systemic digestive or enzyme issues.
- Skin ulcers that do not heal.
- Chronic iron deficiency.
- Elevated histamine responses.
- Contracture of ligaments.
- Endocrine issues. Male and female infertility. Low sperm count.
- Mitochondrial issues, adenosine triphosphate (ATP) issues, glutathione deficiency.
- Encephalitis. Brain cry.
- Hyperactivity, ADHD, and ADD.
- Suppressed immune system, weak immune system.
    - Chronic fatigue syndrome (CFS)
    - History of vaccines.
    - Co-infections:
        - Un-resolving sickness.
        - Herpes, EBV, Cytomegalovirus.
        - Lyme's disease.
        - Hepatitis B.
    - Cancer.

15. Homeopathic Remedies to Repair Glyphosate Damage

For those new to homeopathy, please work with a practitioner.

The remedies discussed below are suggestions in relationship to the pathogenesis of glyphosate toxicity and are not a complete list. A number of these remedies I have confirmed in clinical cases of glyphosate toxicity. The others I have deduced through symptom similarity. Clinical experience will add to the following list. Refer to Materia Medica volumes for specific symptom confirmations.

The rubrics referenced, and associated remedies, are sourced from the Boenninghausen Repertory. While current day repertories may have more complete remedy listings, the size of the rubric is not helpful for the summaries review here. It is my opinion that the remedies listed in Boenninghausen are more clinically verifiable due to their historical confirmation and were sourced at a time when glyphosate toxicity did not confound natural pathology.

While it may look like I am suggesting giving all remedies at once, this not possible. However, clinical experience has taught me you will need to intercurrent with several remedies in different potencies at the same time to make any effect. For example:

- Bowel nosodes: high dose 200, 1M, or higher: weekly or monthly.
- Miasmatic nosodes mid-range potency, 200C: weekly, on Saturday.
- Constitutional remedies: 30C: daily, Monday through Friday.
- Organ specific remedies: low C or X potencies: daily.
- Cell salts: x potencies: daily.
- LMs are not suited for this application.
- **Glyphosate Clearing Protocol** when ready.

Miasmatic Influences (indications for these nosodes):

- ***Psorinum***: A remedy for Psora. Weak recuperative powers with a tendency towards irritation of tissues. Clear, bland, or irritating discharges. Skin, digestive and metabolic disorders, Hypothyroidism. Constipation. Malnutrition and poverty. Gout, from irritation. Lack of motivation to change anything Fear of poverty. The farmer in business, hard-working but feeling like he is failing.
- ***Medorrhinum***: A remedy for sycosis. Tendency towards excessive mucopurulent discharges. Damage to kidneys, gout from hyperexcretion of uric acid. Hyperproliferation of cancer cells. Endometriosis. Greed, gluttony, and obesity. Wanting more, bigger, and better. The capitalist. Prospering by exploiting others.
- ***Syphilinum***: A remedy for syphilitic tendencies. Breakdown in proper collagen formation. Deformities. Suicidal and homicidal tendencies. Progressive degenerative neurological conditions. Neural tube defects. Skin ulcers, endocrine issues, cardiovascular and glandular issues. There is no way out of this hopeless situation. Shutting down to cope. Banker or investor losing all capital.
- ***Tuberculinum***: Tuberculosis, latent or active, sets up allergic and inflammatory responses. ***Tuberculinum*** can help to resolve asthma, hyperthyroidism, wasting diseases, long bones. Hyperactivity, restlessness, and destructive tendencies Hopeful and fighting your way out by mass protest or revolution. The revolutionary, artist, or writer not willing to be imprisoned. The rebel, anarchist, and untamable.
- ***Carcinosin***:* Tendency to cancer, ailments from suppression of the immune system. Food allergies, systemic allergies, asthma, auto-immune conditions, glandular conditions. Co-infections, Lyme's disease, herpes, retroviruses, Epstein-Barr virus (EBV) (glandular fever), cancerous cell proliferation and gene mutations. Insomnia and asthma (adenosine receptor activation and deficiency of adenosine deaminase). Suppression of the individual. Mass production of cloned foods. No individualization, failure to differentiate. Going along with the flow and not wanting to take a stand or stand out. Dominated, controlled, and controlling. Easily

suppressed, fear of the void. Use for deactivation of adenosine receptor sites and removal of immune suppression.
*Note on sources of ***Carcinosin*** (breast cancer): not all sources are the same. The one I use comes from unknown source in India from the 1980's and seems more vitally active that the one sourced from Hahnemann Labs in the US or Helios Pharmacy in the UK. There is also ***Carcinosin co.*** (13 tumors) and ***Carcinosin T58*** (58 tumors). ***Cuprum cum Carcinosin*** is a combination of copper and ***Carcinosin*** for those who are excessively controlled and rigid. Works with acetylcholine receptors to release to contractions, spasms, and cramps. ***Carcinosin*** also works with DNA gene editing managed by zinc dependent adenosine deaminase (ADA), or copper-dependent enzyme amine oxidase (AO) to metabolize adenosine occupying the adenosine receptor sites, or zinc-dependent diamine oxidase (DAO), needed to reduce histamine levels. There is also ***Scirrhinum*** made from a cancerous tumor.

- ***AIDS*** (***Human immunodeficiency virus (HIV)*** nosode): Disintegration of the DNA and collapse of the immune system. Co-infections with multiple viruses otherwise benign infections. Cancer. Failure to sexually differentiate. Radiation. Paranoia, mistrust, and feelings of persecution. Must isolate to protect self from persecution. Distortions in the shape and sizes of erythrocytes.

Overview of Cell Salts:

Homeopathic Cell salts are remedies made from essential minerals that are vital to all cellular functions. Given individually or in series they each support the various functions these minerals perform. While few of these Cell salts specifically address the issues relating to glyphosate toxicity, this does not diminish their effect on general wellbeing and organ function. These remedies can be given as intercurrents to other remedies. Typically to be used in low potency: I prefer 9x. The following remedies can also be used constitutionally if symptoms match.

#1. ***Calcarea fluorica***: Elasticity salt, improves strength of collagen, bones, and teeth. In cases with weak collagen, bones, and teeth. Thyroid conditions, tubercular and syphilitic manifestations. Misappropriation of calcium.

#2. ***Calcarea phosphorica***: General cellular tonic, nutrition salt, bone health, connective tissue formation (collagen). Indicated in adenosine triphosphate (ATP) issues, poor brain development, and calcium channel dysfunction. Feeble digestion, insufficient bile acids, poor stamina, glandular enlargements, iron deficient anemia, bone pains and bone cancer.

#3. ***Calcarea sulphurica***: Cell healer, blood purifier, removal of waste products. In cases of calcium or sulfur deficiency, inability to fully digest sulphurated foods. In instances of low oxygen and disturbed metabolism leading to increased pyruvic acid, lactic acid and other intimidate by products of glycolysis. Tendency towards yellow pustulation and eczema, cystic tumors, hard swellings, and collagen disorders (lax fibers). Removal of old and dysfunctional red or white blood cells, thus is a blood and liver cleanser. Helps bile acid production and emulsification of fats. Helps to prevent kidney- and gallstones.

#4. ***Ferrum phosphorica***: Ferrum (iron) adds to the hemoglobin which is an oxygen carrier: increases oxygen in the blood. ***Phosphorus*** strengthens the blood structure and blood vessels. To help build the blood by increasing both iron and phosphorus. Supports the immune system, maintains and builds fevers. Use to carry the fever through infective processes. Vitamin C increases functionally of ***Ferrum phosphoricum.***

#5. ***Kali muriaticum***: Blood purifier, heart tonic, and glandular tonic. Helps to clear thick white fibrinous discharges. Subacute inflammatory conditions. Potassium (kali) calms the sympathetic nervous system and blood plasma potassium concentrations. Helps to reduce swelling.

#6. ***Kali phosphoricum***: Nerve nutrient, counteracts weakness and decay, activates cellular energy (Krebs cycle). Facilities the creation of nucleic acids (DNA and RNA) and utilization of the energy compounds: ATP, ADP, and AMP. Without potassium phosphate increased acidosis occurs. Weakness and exhaustion leading to over-excitability and nervous dread. Want of nerve power, prostration. Disturbance in the sympathetic nervous system. Adynamia and decay, malignant tumors.

#7. ***Kali sulphuricum***: Skin balance, helps carry oxygen to cells for all oxidative processes. It is also used in the formation of collagen in connective tissue and skin. Profuse desquamation. Later stages of inflammation (when oxygen levels are low) in cases marked by excessive yellow discharge due to lack of oxygen. Damage from calcium oxalate and kidney stones, end stage renal disease. Psoriasis, nettle rash (urticaria).

#8. ***Magnesium phosphorica***: Nerve relaxant, anti-spasmodic salt, reduces cramps and spasmodic activity. In cases of poor intestinal motility. Tiered and exhausted, nerve pains in the teeth, ears, muscles, intestines, headaches. Bloating, indigestion, intestines full of gas causing colic. Tics and spasms. Deficiency of magnesium phosphate induces increased calcium levels and an increase in 'bad' cholesterol causing hardening, plaques, the tendency towards kidney stones and cardiac arrest. ***Magnesium phosphorica*** will facilitate the deposit of calcium back in the bones. It reduces spasticity by reducing acetylcholine levels and resultant deactivation of the nicotinic acetylcholine receptors (nAChRs).

#9. ***Natrum muriaticum***: Fluid balancer, water distribution of salt. In cases of headaches from liver stagnation. Anemia from iron deficiency, leukocytosis, edema. Retention of fluids, and metabolites creating rheumatic gout. Hyperthyroidism, Addison's disease, diabetes. Weakness and old grief. Constant feeling of coldness.

#10. ***Natrum phosphoricum***: Acid neutralizer, lactic acid converter, release of cellular water to extracellular space for urination or weeping. ***Natrum phosphoricum*** releases hydrogen (H^+) rendering the system more alkaline: it serves as a pH balancer.

Emulsifies fatty acids leading to production of bile acids. Reduces gallstones and gout. Helps to establish healthy biome and reduce excess lactic acid from consumption of too much sugar. Yellow creamy coated tongue, lump in the throat, jaundice, and sour belching. Colic, leukorrhea and infertility by the system being too acidic and killing the sperm. Worms due to purification of proteins, ammonia, and carbon dioxide in the intestines. Lactic acidosis and high oxalates in the urine. Helps to release old grief held in the heart.

#11. ***Natrum sulphuricum***: Normalizes the blood, bile and pancreatic juices by increasing oxygen. Facilitates the release of water from cellular respiration (glycolysis). Reduces lactic acid to carbonic acid and water. Water eliminator from extracellular space and brain , liver detoxifier by promoting the free flow of bile. In cases of liver insufficiency, or insufficient bile. Natrum sulfate is a constituent of healthy collagen, promoting elasticity. Facilitates absorption of calcium. It is also present in vitamins (thiamine (B1), biotin (B7), etc.), amino acids (methionine, homocysteine, cysteine, and glutathione), hormones, insulin, enzymes, and coenzymes. It helps to reduce the phenol groups from the metabolism of phenylalanine, tyrosine, and tryptophan. For diabetes and high cholesterol. Thick discharges. Expels worms.

#12. ***Silicea***: Cell cleanser, nutrient to all cells, detoxifier, and general immune system stimulant. Stimulates phagocytosis. By increasing neutrophils and macrophages. Activates immune response to *Streptococcus* and *Staphylococcus* bacteria by facilitating the release of pus (the general immune system response generated by macrophage phagocytosis of these bacteria). Helps absorb calcium and fluorine. To help detox aluminum and support nutritional absorption. Imperfect assimilation of nutrients, abscesses, wounds that do not heal, too cold, and does not recover from acute illnesses. Stimulates white blood cell activity and suppurative processes. Easily overstimulated nerves, sensitive to environmental stimuli. Rousts recuperative powers.

Focus of Homeopathic Treatment in Order of Priority:

This section mirrors chapter 10. Summary: Absorption Routes and Complications of Glyphosate. Prioritize which pathogenesis of glyphosate toxicity you want to address first with related remedies. Work through the layers and prioritize as to most limiting expression to constitutional work. What I have also seen is well indicated remedies will fail to act as the operator of glyphosate continues to maintain the diseased symptom expression. To address long-term issues, it is better to give low potency over several weeks (considered nutritional dosing) than try a single dose high potency prescription (energetic dosing).

I. Biome and Intestinal Lining:

Homeopathic Philosophy on Bacterial Balance: The conventional view of bacteria, especially of those bacteria that are present in pathological conditions, is to blame the bacteria for the sickness. As a result, the conventional mindset is to use antibiotics to kill the bacteria that are present in these pathological processes. The problem is that antibiotics kill all commensal bacteria as well and force pathological bacteria to develop antibiotic resistance. Supplementation with probiotics can help to restore the healthy bacteria, however, this alone will not change the pathological environment that was conducive for the respective bacteria to grow in the first place. That environment is a condition of the individual and only energetic changes produced by remedies can address this.

The homeopathic point of view is that bacteria mutate and become pathological when the system is out of balance, e.g. when the individual becomes sick, either through errors in living or environmental exposures, that weaken the system (too much heat, cold, work, stress, or otherwise). The energetic matrix of the system maintains balance or discord. By addressing the energetic issues that set the system out of balance with homeopathic remedies, the symptom manifestation, e.g. the bacterial imbalance, should correct itself. If it does not, then, nosodes (homeopathic remedies made from pathological cultures (bacteria) or diseased tissue) are used to reorganize the system that sets up the environment that was conducive to propagating the respective bacteria. Accordingly, when the symptom presentation of the individual manifests as *Streptococcal* disease, *Candida* overgrowth, *Salmonella,* or *Clostridium difficile* disease, for example, rather than giving medicines aimed at killing these disease agents, e.g. antibiotics or antifungals, we give homeopathic preparations of these same agents to ask the system to resolve the energetic imbalance that allowed for the propagation of those bacteria to begin with. Rife machines work on this same principle.

The symptom pictures presented below are the indications for the remedy and should be matched with the symptoms of the person. In cases of glyphosate toxicity, as the natural biome is severely disturbed, vigilance to restoring bacterial balance is necessary. Doses of these nosodes may need to be repeated often and maintained throughout the detox process especially if there is continued glyphosate exposure, in addition to supplemental probiotics to rebuild the healthy populations.

The resultant effect of giving bacterial nosodes may be to stimulate an exonerative diarrhea to rid the offending populations, or a fever to normalize the immune system response to the normally commensal bacteria. These effects should not be mitigated unless they do not resolve on their own. If they do not resolve, treat with other homeopathic remedies based on symptom presentation to continue the process towards normalization. Nosodes can be alternated with the symptom specific remedies. Homeopathic repair of the intestinal lining must be accompanied by dietary changes.

The problem of an unestablished healthy biome comes in children that were born while the mother was on antibiotics, or if she did not have a healthy biome in the first place. The intestinal lining of these children never properly developed. In these instances, the job of the homeopath becomes more complex and greater vigilance is needed to help establish and maintain a healthy biome and the appropriate tight junction gaps of the intestinal lining for clear thinking and discernment. As the biome is the root of developmental processes, hormonal regulation, and neurological development, this work is ever more paramount for children with pervasive developmental delays.

Remedies to Address the Biome and Intestinal Lining:

Liquor amnii, AKA ***Aqua amniotica***: For infants, as a healthy biome is first established by healthy amniotic fluid in utero, it makes sense that the reestablishment of the intestinal biome could first be addressed by this amazing remedy. This is the original cell salt we are bathed in. It is indicated by a feeling of something missing, something unresolved, a longing to go back to something, of being lost, even abandoned. Wanting to go back to the ocean and breathe underwater. A sense of control to protect one-self from being hurt again or abandoned. A feeling of vulnerability and vigilance to protect oneself. Deep grief. Collective grief for humanity and the Mother Earth. Consider aqua marina if the infant's biome never established a relationship with *Lactobacillus* bacteria. Much like ***Natrum muriaticum*** or ***Aqua marina*** but more complex due to the added trace mineral content. In addition to the salts, urea, proteins, and carbohydrates found in the fluid, varying concentrations of fifteen other minerals and trace elements have been measured: aluminum, arsenic, calcium, chromium, cobalt, copper, iron, lead, magnesium, nickel, potassium, rubidium, selenium, silver, strontium, and zinc. Consider anyone of these minerals as remedies based on symptom expression.

Aqua marina: Made from ocean water, consists of minerals required by our genetic code: sodium, magnesium, calcium, potassium, strontium, chlorine, sulfite, carbonate, bromine, borate, iodine, fluorine, aluminum and iron oxides, silica, and a number of other trace minerals. The pH of sea water is maintained at 8.0–8.4 by a buffering system. Because the water is alkaline, most of the calcium and hydrogen carbonate form insoluble calcium carbonate (CaCO3). From this alkaline environment, most living organisms have their origin: the primordial sea. Correspondingly, ***Aqua marina*** is a fundamental remedy for maintaining well-being in the entire body: cardiovascular, nervous and endocrine systems, metabolism, creation of bile salts, preservation of cellular integrity, and alkalinity of the body. In cases of old grief, delusions they have done wrong and been wronged. Suppressed emotional storms: would rather not speak for fear of losing composure, but rage, grief, and delusions of being hard-done-by can overwhelm the emotional body. Remains calm on the exterior. Helps to normalize hyper- and hypothyroidism and adrenal function (excess cortisol). When some or many of the single elements are indicated think of ***Aqua marina***. It matches the silent grief of ***Natrum muriaticum***, which, however, is experienced like an internal typhoon. Reserved, and doesn't want people looking at them. Ailments from being observed.

Polio nosode: a remedy for tight junction issues. A remedy for control, fear, and the inability to stand up and defend yourself. Feeling of being overwhelmed by external forces. Lack of ability to discern what is good for you or not. If you can imagine that the tight junctions of the intestinal lining not properly gated, e.g. an upregulation of zonulin, you can image the experience of the spleen trying to filter the circulatory system overburdened by undigested food stuff and pathogenic material trafficked across the intestinal lining. These open tight junctions lead to stimulation of the vagus nerve and an over reactive fight or flight response resulting in inability to rationally sort through life's events, ushering in the possibility of becoming easily dominated, suppressed, and surrendering your individuality to the control of others. Consider ***Polio*** to close those tight junctions and bring order to the immune system. What needs to be eliminated and what needs to be adsorbed? Who am I and who am I not?

Injection of the inactivated polio virus vaccine (IPV), rather than greater auto-regulatory powers, the potential benefits produced by oral exposure to wild virus, the immune system becomes more susceptible to dysregulation.[cxlii] This phenomena, instigated by the global polio eradication vaccination program, beginning in the late 1950's early 1960's, nearly every person on the planet was affected. The result of which is varying degrees of fear, oppression, lack of discernment, and a form of paralysis against/or compliance to patriarchal and global power structures. Moreover, as early vaccines were incubated on mouse serum mediums, they became contaminated with the RNA retrovirus, xenotropic murine leukemia virus (XMRV). This virus has been associated with weakness, muscle pain, impaired memory and/or mental concentration, and post-exertional fatigue, insomnia, and chronic fatigue syndrome. Research has demonstrated that XMRV has contaminated inactivated polio vaccines compounding auto-immune dysregulation.[cxliii] Consider remedies that can treat polio and affect the acetylcholine receptor sites for associated effects: ***Lathyrus sativus***, ***Physostigma***, ***Nux vomica***, ***Gelsemium***,, ***Hydrocyanic acid***, ***Laurocerasus***, ***Curare***, etc.

Natrum phosphoricum: The main remedy to address a hyper acidic environment. Use to normalize pH balance. Too much sugar or insufficient blood oxygen can lead to excess lactic acid and the subsequent conditions arising from intestinal acidosis. Lacto-fermenting bacteria are necessary to all metabolic processes however, deficiency in the molybdenum dependent enzymes needed to metabolize the lactic acid can lead to excess, resulting in small intestinal bacterial overgrowth (SIBO) or hyper histamine activity and *Candida*. Use ***Natrum phosphoricum*** to facilitate a change in internal pH imbalance from acidic to alkaline. It affects the duodenum, bile ducts. Conversely, ***Natrum phosphoricum*** will also help to restore acidity to the vaginal biome. Sour belching and taste, sour vomiting. Inflammation of the back of the throat. Worms, colic, jaundice, cerebral inflammation. Excessive histamine levels from too much lactic acid also lactic acidosis driven cerebral inflammation. ***Natrum phosphoricum*** facilitates the metabolism of lactic acid to carbonic acid which is then liberated through the lungs in exchange for oxygen. Increased oxygen decreases acidity. Vinegar can also convert excess lactic acid to lactate then to carbon dioxide and water. See: IX. **Endocrine System** below for hormonal drivers of excess histamine. See X. **Immune System** for immunological drivers of excess histamine.

Rheum – Rhubarb: a remedy often needed in young children with irritable temperament, colic, and sour stools. It is useful to reset intestinal pH.

Torula cervisiae – *Saccharomyces cervisiae* (and *Saccharomyces boulardi*) are types of yeast that help to reduce specific bacterial populations that can lead to inflammation due to excess lactic acid levels. This remedy is indicated in conditions of systemic allergic eczema, anaphylaxis states produced by the inability to digest proteins and more specifically in conditions where there is a lack of trypsin (e.g. deficient *Bifidobacteria* needed for the creation of trypsin (lacto-fermenting bacteria)). *Saccharomyces boulardi* is recommended as a supplement to reduce lactic acid and excess histamine. ***Torula cervisiae*** is to address the physical manifestations outlined above. Note: the hepatitis B vaccine is incubated on *Saccharomyces cervisiae*. The same conditions created by the yeast are present in vaccine damage from the hepatitis B vaccine. Vaccine detox may be necessary to resolve this condition.

Candida albicans or ***parapsilosis*** – *Candida albicans/parapsilosis*: (one can purchase a single remedy or combination of the two). Overgrowth is demonstrated by brain fog, sugar cravings, laughing, hyperactivity, skin rashes, clusters of small red pin-sized spots (especially around the mouth, vagina, or anus, under the breasts, underarms, and groin area (warm and moist areas)). Fermented stools, constipation, mucus in stools, bloating, undigested stools, or floating stools. Laughing, giggling, stupefaction, and retardation. Worse from beer and mold exposure. Intercurrent ***Candida*** in cases of iron deficiency, recurrent *Streptococcal* fevers, and insufficient fevers. When reducing yeast populations, it is normal for fevers to arise so as to keep rising bacteria populations in check. For instance, *Streptococc*us bacteria should normally be present in the body. When you lower yeast with ***Candida***, *streptococcus* bacteria will normally reestablish itself. However, a fever might come in which case you need to give ***Streptococcinum*** or ***Staphylococcinum*** –*Staphylococcus* bacteria: to help keep this insurgent population in check. When fevers come, treat with homeopathic remedies that match the symptom presentation of those fevers. After administration, changes in bowel function are normal and expected as the system discharges the excess *Candida*. Systemic *Candida* conditions, ones where the *Candida* is in the blood stream and liver (demonstrated by toe nail fungus (large toe corresponds to the liver, fungus here indicates yeast in the liver)) will take longer to clear. Use ascending potencies as needed. It takes 3 months for the toe nails to grow out clear and about as long to rid the system. Intercurrent with ***Natrum phosphoricum*** to address the acid issues, and ***Ferrum phosphoricum*** for iron issues and to build the blood to carry the fevers necessary to balance the repopulation of commensal bacteria. Eliminate all sugar from the diet.

Streptococcinum –*Streptococcus pyogenes* (or other multiple variant species) or ***Scarlatinum*** (historical dose discharge of scarlet fever): may be needed to normalize naturally occurring lacto-fermenting *Streptococcal* bacteria that will proliferate once the *Candida* population is lowered. Use ***Belladonna***, ***Hepar sulphuris calcareum***, or ***Phytolacca***, for example, or others, to treat the symptoms produced when the immune system is working to develop a balance with *Streptococcus* bacteria (sore throat, deposits in the throat, swollen glands, fevers, bad breath, nausea, headache, etc.). These remedies do not kill the *Streptococcal* bacteria but rather help normalize the individual's relationship to the bacteria. There is a misunderstanding that the culturing of *Streptococcus* means that it is responsible for the symptoms present. More often antibiotics are prescribed only for the fever to return once the course of antibiotics have finished. PANDAS (Pediatric Auto-immune Neuropsychiatric Disorders Associated with *Streptococcal* Infections) is a condition that arises from the immune system over-reacting to *Streptococcus* bacteria. If antibiotics are given repeatedly the immune system will remain in a state whereby it is trying to keep the bacteria in check or will let the yeast colonize the entire body (sweet or alcohol smelling breath will tell you this is so). The bacteria are not the problem, rather it is the condition of the individual.

Staphylococcinum, and/or ***MRSA nosode***: may be needed: *Methicillin-resistant Staphylococcus aureus (MRSA)* is glyphosate resistant and will naturally populate in an individual with glyphosate toxicity. Indicated in ulcerating skin infections. Impetigo, necrosis, and hemolysis. Alternate with ***Candida albicans*** as needed.

Clostridium difficile – *Clostridium difficile:* impedes the conversion of dopamine to norepinephrine and epinephrine due to reduction in the enzyme tyrosine hydroxylase. Cases of severe addictive behavior (excessive dopamine), isolation, or schizophrenia may have *Clostridium difficile* as the root cause. *Clostridium difficile* overgrowth activates (is an agonist to*) the nicotinic acetylcholine receptor sites (nAChRs) in the intestines resulting in alternating constipation and diarrhea, or frequent diarrhea (3-15 times a day), ulcerative colitis, intestinal pain, licking the lips, cerebral inflammation, distress, head banging, hitting, and biting behavior. In potency ***Clostridium difficile*** releases these same sites and expels the bacteria in the stool. Nicotine is an antagonist* (means turns off the site) to the *C-difficile* toxin indicating nicotine as a preventive to toxicity from *clostridium difficile* while not changing the active population. This means a smoker may harbor *clostridium difficile* without active disease symptoms. ***Tabacum*** is indicated in prostration, profuse vomiting and diarrhea, pallor, increased perspiration and salivation, indicating the muscarinic receptors are also involved with this remedy. ***Podophyllum***, in long standing diarrhea with cerebral inflammation. ***Jaborandi***, contains pilocarpine, in hot flushes, nausea, diarrhea, salivation, and profuse perspiration. Other remedies in the *Clostridium* family as nosodes (***C. tetani***, ***C. botulin***) may also be indicated by their associated symptoms presentation. The toxin of *C. tetani* produces spastic paralysis and exaggerated tendon reflexes and is Zinc dependent (consider ***C. tetani*** or ***Zincum***). Remedies in the Solanaceae family: ***Belladonna***, ***Stramonium***, or ***Hyoscyamus*** may be indicated as they are also antagonists in crude doses to these sites. Cerebral inflammation causes a kind of shrieking called brain cry or cri encephalique. It is characterized by a high pitch whining or whaling sound and sometimes rolling of the head, boring it into the pillow, or banging of the head. It is often accompanied by teeth grinding. This symptom presentation is common to these remedies.

Antagonistic or agonistic action and homeopathy**: In homeopathy selection of remedies is based on symptom presentation and matching the symptoms of the person to those of the human reaction to the toxic or crude dose of the same substance. In crude dose each substance has a primary action, while in potency, often the opposite action is stimulated. This means that in potency you can release the action of an agonist. The isopathic approach is giving the exact same substance as this which causes the toxicity, e.g. using ***Clostridium difficile. Thus, the primary action of *clostridium difficile* is agonistic to the nicotinic acetylcholine receptor sites (nAChRs), and in potency the reverse affect will be true. The homeopathic approach is to use another substance that produces a similar symptom presentation. Crude Belladonna matches the symptom profile and atropine acts as an antagonist to acetylcholine receptors (means deactivates) thus, in potency, ***Belladonna*** can address this symptom presentation as well. Others listed in the follow rubric may be indicated:

Mind; Shrieking**,** screaming, shouting; brain: ***Aml-n.***, **APIS**, arn., ars., ***Art-v.***, bell., bor., bry., calc., calc-hp., canth., ***Carb-ac.***, ***Cham.***, cic., ***Cina***, coff., crot-c., **CUPR***.,* ***Cupr-acet.***, cupr-ar., cypr., dig., dpt, dulc., gels., ***Glon.***, ***Hell.***, ***Hyos.***, ign., iodof., ***Kali-br.***, ***Kali-i.***, lac-h., ***Lyc.***, merc., merc-c., merc-v., nat-p., nux-m., per., phos., plb., ***Rhus-t.***, ***Sol-n.***, ***Solin.***, stram., sulph., syph., tub., verat-v. ***Zincum***, and ***Brass*** also.

Pseudomonas variants: This primitive species co-propagates with *Clostridium difficile* as an adaptive mechanism by synthesizing cholinesterase. This serves to deactivate the acetylcholine receptors *C. diff* toxins activate. To ensure their survival in the intestines they create biofilms from the cellular lining of the intestines producing "rope worms." *Pseudomonas* species can be impacted by the mineral gallium. Although gallium has no natural function in biology, gallium ions interact with cellular processes in a manner similar to iron$^{(+3)}$. When gallium ions are mistakenly taken up in place of iron$^{(+3)}$ by *Pseudomonas*, the ions interfere with respiration, and they die. Thus, ***Gallium*** may be used homeopathically in cases of *Pseudomonas*. Proving symptoms include: 'I had to dive into it, drown in its frozen waters, swim with its crabs, and fly with its crows. It took me on a voyage of birth and death, and to the limbo in between, to tidal waves, floods, strife, civil war, the dawn of mankind and its Armageddon, but also to healing, care, and resolution. Of great value in post-traumatic stress disorder, severe grief and depression, its possible use as a resurrector from sudden traumatic death' (Jeremey Sherr). This reminds one of the primordial seas, and the source from which the entire biome is established. By addressing the *Clostridium* populations, *Pseudomonas* species will naturally decline.

Bowel nosodes: Remedies made from non-lacto-fermenting bacteria which are a part of the normal intestinal biome. That which, when the system is under stress, specific strains propagate and monopolize the system. Bowel nosodes are used to bring the biome back into balance and facilitate the shedding of over-grown populations.

Sycotic co. – *Neisseria mucosa* – or *Streptococcus faecalis* (original identification of sources for this nosode are conflicting siding more with *Neisseria – Gonorrhea*). Originating in sycosis. Consider also ***Medorrhinum***. Chronic gastric irritation, rectal prolapse. Pale waxy skin, Asthma.

Dysenteriae co. – *Shigella*: Nervous, restless, and apprehensive. Chronic indigestion, loose bowels, ulcers.

Mutabilis – The bacterial intermediary between *Coli bacilli* and *Lactobacillus*. It mutates based on the environment: may be indicated to help stabilize *Escherichia* bacterial populations (*E. coli*). Alternating skin eruptions and asthmatic symptoms. Cystitis and malnutrition. Sallow complexion.

Bacillus #7 – *Enterobacter cloacae asiaticus freuni*: Worn out, great mental and physical weakness. Prematurely old, feeble. Light sleep. Can't digest fats. Constipation and hemorrhoids. Eructations. Pale and cold.

Gaertner – *Salmonella*: Malnutrition, diarrhea, bites nails, hypersensitive over-active brain, gallstones, bloody stools, nausea, excessive eructation, indigestion, antibiotic poisoning. Restlessness, excitable and depressed, worms. *Salmonella* is present in undercooked chicken, on the surface of eggs. ***Typhoidium*** is *Salmonella typhi*, this can lead to severe watery stools, intestinal hemorrhage, bleeding beneath the skin, septic conditions, and coma.

Proteus – *Enterobacteria* indicated by brainstorm fits of temper, irritable from nervous strain. Rectal spasm, peptic ulcers, alternating diarrhea and constipation, bleeding hemorrhoids. Allergic conditions, food sensitivities, digestive allergies, acrid dyspepsia. Pinworms.

Morgan – From non-lacto-fermenting bacteria. Congestion and inflammation: Irritable and depressed, hepatic congestion, headaches with red face. Itching skin with purulent eruptions. Constipation. Biliary lithiasis (gallstones), inflammation of the gallbladder. Sulfur issues, CYP protein enzyme deficiency and insufficient cholesterin. Consider in MTHFR gene mutations.

Motility issues (constipation):

- **Insufficient bile**: in this order; ***Lycopodium***, ***Chelidonium***, ***Colocynthis***, ***Phosphorus***, ***Sulphur***, ***Pulsatilla***, ***Sepia***, ***Natrum muriaticum***, ***Opium***.
- **Calcium channel issues** (defective myosin contraction) leading to constipation: ***Calcarea carbonica***, ***Calcarea phosphorica***, ***Silicea***, ***Sanicula*** (spring water with many trace minerals).

Remedy dosing: As ***candida*** overgrowth in the intestines is the main outcome of glyphosate toxicity its normalization is primary to addressing the biome. Listed below is suggested dosing for four weeks while the client is cleaning out their cupboards and beginning nutritional detox. Supportive probiotics and collagen supplementation can be started. These remedies can be given concurrently with each other and with constitutional prescribing. Use this for the first month of treatment. Reassess continuation based on reaction and new symptoms presenting before moving to the next phase. *Note: nosodes are given in high potency successively according to the days noted. Give constitutional after nosodes, to maximize duration of action before next dose of nosode.

According to the chart on the next page give ***Candida*** before ***Streptococcinum*** or bowel nosodes. Alternate ***Streptococcinum*** with ***Clostridium difficile*** or ***Staphylococcinum*** as needed, based on symptoms (e.g. sore throat, acetylcholine activation symptoms, or impetigo respectively). If the fevers are insufficient or there is systemic *Candida,* dose with ***Ferrum phosphoricum*** for several weeks to build the iron sources and the blood so as to get the sufficient fever. Treat surfacing conditions with nutritional or mechanical support (salt water gargle), or with more specific symptom-indicated remedies. I.e. ***Argentum nitricum*** of ***Lycopodium*** for *Candida* (gas, bloating, sugar cravings etc.), ***Belladonna*** or ***Hepar sulphuris calcareum*** for *Streptococcus* infections, ***Apis*** or ***Calendula*** for *Staphylococcus* infections, etc.

	Remedy	When Concurrent dosing	Duration
1	***Natrum phosphoricum*** 9x	Monday - Friday. To increase pH and lower lactic acid.	4 weeks in a.m.
2	***Candida*** 30C or 200C*	Wednesday and Saturday. Or each Saturday.	4 weeks in p.m.
3 **or**	***Streptococcinum*** 1M*	Sunday.	4 weeks.
3	Bowel nosode or ***Clostridium difficile*** 200C* or 1M*	Sunday.	4 weeks.
4	Constitutional remedy.	Monday 200C* or Monday - Friday 30C.	4 weeks in p.m.
5	H/O suppressed fevers, insufficient fevers, or iron deficiency: ***Ferrum phosphoricum*** *9x* .	Monday - Friday.	4 weeks at noon if needed.
	Repeat cycle if necessary		

II. Nutritional Deficiencies:

One must ask, is the nutritional deficiency due to lack of nutrients, lack of absorption, deficient enzymes needed to reduce or oxidize the food, or leaching of essential minerals? From a vitalism point of view (homeopathic philosophy) you can address deficiencies energetically with remedies despite nutritional deficiencies within a certain range. The energetic information from the remedy serves to reestablish the body's relationship with the relative mineral so that it is more easily maintained within the body. This shows itself either through absorption or cessation of leaching.

Granted, one does need vital nutrients in the food we eat, but sometimes, no matter the nutrient density of food consumed, the body does not take up the nutrient, or despite supplementation the nutrient is still leached from the body. Absorption is based on pH levels, relative oxygen levels, and functionality of enzymes and the transmembrane channels of the cells that would take up the nutrients. The blueprint registering the kind of environment needed to maintain appropriate nutrition is held in the memory of the DNA. The factor governing the ability for the DNA to transcribe its needs is held in the energetic quality of the system. Homeopathic remedies positively affect the energetics so that the system is aligned to maintain appropriate mineral levels. The main nutrients affected are: sulfur, iron, calcium, manganese, molybdenum, zinc, cobalt, copper, and selenium. The following list of remedies does not cover all nutritional deficits but rather focuses on those specific to glyphosate toxicity.

Generalities; Marasmus: *alum.*, arg., *ars.*, *bar-c.*, calc., calc-p., *carb-an.*, *carb-v.*, caust., *chin.*, con., gaert, graph., helo., *hydr.*, *iod.*, *kali-bi.*, kali-i., kreos., **Lyc.**, mang., *merc.*, mur-ac., nat-m., *nit-ac.*, petr., phos., plb., pyrog., sel., sep., sil., stann., staph., *sulph.*, zinc.

a. **Sulfur deficiency**: Sulfur helps to carry the oxygen for oxidative purposes. It is the basis of methionine and glutathione, and is central in the results of MTHFR gene mutations and methylation issues, enzyme dysfunction with regards to the quaternary structure of proteins (reduction of the sulfur bonds) and inability to metabolize foods high in sulfur: eggs, fish, meat, bone broth, cheese, nuts, legumes, cruciferous vegetables, onions and garlic, peaches, apricots, beer, and foods preserved with sulfites (wine and dried fruit): According to symptom presentations consider ***Sulphur***, ***Kali sulphuricum***, ***Calcarea sulphurica***, ***Hepar sulphuris calcareum***, ***Ammonium sulphuricum***, and the plant remedies high in sulfur: ***Lycopodium***, ***Pulsatilla***, ***Chamomilla***, ***Rumex***, ***Hydrastis***, ***Echinacea***, ***Allium cepa***, and many others that produce some variation of skin complaints, intestinal irritation, constipation or diarrhea, thick yellow mucus, detoxification issues, uric acid diathesis, flatulence and many other conditions.

b. **Iron deficiency**: Deficient iron leads to a host of immune system challenges, reduction in hemoglobin and erythropoietin, all necessary for healthy immune system function. Heme-dependent CYP proteins and enzymes drive the neurulation process and the production of thyroid hormones. Heavy metals change the oxidation levels of iron, compound sedimentation rates, and lower the oxygen carrying capacity of erythrocytes. Consider ***Pulsatilla***, ***Arnica***, ***Natrum muriaticum***, ***Ferrum metallicum***, ***Ferrum muriaticum***, ***Ferrum phosphoricum***, ***Kali sulphuricum***, or other remedies based on relative symptoms. To build the blood suggested dosing is to start ***Ferrum phosphoricum*** 9x Monday to Friday, for two to three weeks and retest. Other remedies as indicated will help the bones make the blood and carry the oxygen. For severe anemia associated with leukemia and swollen spleen – ***Ceanothus*** – 12C or 30C daily Monday to Friday for four-six weeks. Alternate remedies as needed. Night sweats are a common symptom of anemia and are intended to pull on the bones to make more red blood cells. ***Tuberculinum*** is indicated by night sweats. ***Silicea*** or ***Sanicula*** for defective nutritional adsorption. ***Acetic acid*** - Vinegar; for severe anemia, end stage cancer, anemia, acid reflux, emaciation, and profuse night sweats.

c. **Calcium deficiency**: Calcium is vital for enzymatic and DNA regulation of neurulation of the spinal tube in embryonic development. GPCR and calcium channels function in relation to hormone and neurotransmitter intercellular communications. Calcium channels also govern myosin contraction in smooth muscle tissue such as venule contraction in the circulatory system, intestines, gallbladder, heart, and uterus. Calcitonin, a calcium bound protein, helps to lower calcium and phosphate levels by driving them back into the bones or to be excreted via urination. It also helps to metabolize phosphates. Misappropriation of calcium in the form of osteoporosis, gallstones, or kidney stones is an issue with calcium regulation. Calcium and magnesium alternately, enable muscle contraction and relaxation. Calcium also plays an important role in regulation of the thyroid and blood pressure.

The main remedy to think of here is ***Calcarea carbonica*** (calcium carbonate) which is indicated in dysfunction of any and all of the above-mentioned systems and functions. ***Calcarea carbonica***, derived from oyster shells, is important when we consider that evolution of more complex organisms have arisen from those like the Mollusks: simple life forms with basic nervous systems, hormonal, reproductive, and gastrointestinal systems that are governed by the same neurotransmitters, hormones, and metal bound GPCR sites our system uses. All this protected by a calcium carbonate shell (and other trace minerals). In homeopathic potency it has a profound effect on rudimentary contractile systems, nervous, hormonal and gastrointestinal systems. The simplicity of the oyster and all the functions that calcium plays in its existence is not lost in the more complex human animal. Calcium is vital to the functioning of every system. Thus, ***Calcarea carbonica*** is a remedy vital to life and the correction of any imbalance relating to calcium. Eating oysters, well known as aphrodisiacs, have an instantaneous ability to roust one's vital force and increase the functioning of choline and deactivation of the nicotinic acetylcholine receptors (nAChRs). Consider ***Calcarea phosphorica*** with relation to deficient cellular respiration and subsequent lack of ATP (energy), slow bone formation or loss of calcium, bone cancer, and developmental delays with regards to bone and teeth formation.

e. **Metals, Calcium Channels, and GPCR functionality**. Review the various functions of these receptors as compared to the persons symptom presentation and consider the following remedies: ***Cobaltum***, ***Cuprum***, ***Ferrum metallicum***, ***Iodatum***, ***Manganum***, ***Molybdenum***, ***Selenium***, ***Stannum***, and ***Zincum*** as mineral deficiency in any one of these minerals may be a constitutional issue (means that the reason there is a deficiency has to do with the vital force of the individual and their relation to the mineral rather than nutritional deficit). Match symptoms of the patient to associated Materia Medica. Translating symptomatology with the back drop of enzymatic and receptor site processes these minerals are responsible for will serve to give a greater comprehension to their healing potential. For examples, as manganese and/or cobalt supplementation increases iron levels, it would also follow that they would increase oxygenation, which would lower acidity levels. As manganese causes anemia with destruction of the red corpuscles, ***Manganum*** would quickly set things right. Cobalt helps in the repair of myelin in the brain.

f. **Copper and Zinc Ratios**: Biochemical responsibilities associated with zinc include:
   - Enzyme functionality.
   - Nucleic acid metabolism required for the necessary coding of DNA and a series of physiological processes.
   - Cell signaling most importantly designed to defend the body from both real and perceived threats.
   - Apoptosis, referred to as programmed cellular death.

   Zinc is required for the following physiological tasks:
   - Growth and development.
   - Fat metabolism which in most simplistic terms can be thought of as necessary fat storage for energy and support in cells.
   - Brain function.
   - Immune system regulation.

   Copper is responsible for enzyme functionally, metabolism of carbohydrates, production of norepinephrine and the regulation of anxiety (fight or flight responses). Copper and zinc work as antagonists to each other to regulate all systems in the body. Consider ***Brass*** to normalize the ratio between copper and zinc when both ***Cuprum*** and ***Zincum*** symptoms are present (tics, contractions and spasms, or retrocession and regression respectively), in addition to all symptoms related to acetylcholine (ACh) receptor site activation (copper and zinc dependent). And to regulate the enzymes amine oxidase (AO) (copper dependent) and diamine oxidase (DAO) (zinc or cobalt activated, copper inhibited). ***Cuprum*** is the rule follower, dictator, and maintains fixed ideas. While this presentation may seem pathological, it is vitally important in DNA replication and immune system regulation (amine oxidase (AO) activity), thus the ***Cuprum*** state is one where the individual is attempting to maintaining their internal order. Conversely, the ***Zincum*** state is marked by repetition, regression, and retrocession, zinc deficiency leads to histamine inflammatory states, which when occurring in the brain is marked by neurological and cognitive regression, learning difficulties, and poor memory. Zinc nourishes the left side of the brain where verbal skills and learning take place. Insufficiency of zinc leads to inability to learn while too much can lead to over analytical/under compassionate qualities (Asperger syndrome). Copper regulates the side of the brain which governs healthy social and tribal qualities. It also governs the truth in the gene editing process in DNA replication. Copper toxicity can lead to rigidity, control, and violence. ***Brass*** would be indicated to help regulate and normalize copper/zinc ratios and right/left brain balance. ***Cuprum*** or ***Zincum*** individually would be indicated if either side of the brain dysfunctional seems more dominant.

III. Enzymes:

Many digestive enzymes are produced by healthy gut biome from the precursor phenylalanine. Others come from live foods. The rest are secreted from cells along the digestive tract, starting in the mouth by the salivary glands, stomach, pancreas, and small intestines. Insufficient enzymes leads to non-digestion of food.

a. Dysbiosis leads to fermentation rather that oxidation of sugars and fats through the Krebs cycle. The main remedies indicated for fermentation/enzymatic deficiency from disturbance in gut biome would be ***Carbo vegetabilis***, ***Lycopodium***, ***China***, ***Argentum nitricum*** (all remedies with belching, bloating, or sugar issues (*Candida* overgrowth). Consider ***Candida***.
b. For CYP protein driven enzymatic dysfunction consider ***Ferrum*** or ***Sulphur*** based remedies as most CYP proteins are either heme- or sulfur- dependent.
c. NAD^{++} deficiency is driven by lactic acidosis. Fast and consider ***Natrum phosphoricum***..
d. The enzyme diamine oxidase (DAO) (for oxidation of histamine) in inhibited in increased concentrations of copper, and activated by zinc to function in its methylation of excess histamine. Consider ***Cuprum*** or ***Zincum***, to regulate functionality, or the

typical antihistamine remedies such as ***Apis***, ***Histaminum***, ***Fragaria***, ***Urtica urens***, or ***Arsenicum***.

e. Elevated histamine in the brain requires the enzyme histamine-N-methyltransferase (dependent upon the *E. coli* synthesis of S-adenosylmethionine (SAM) for its production). Consider ***Mutabilis*** *I (E. coli* bowel nosode) to normalize *E. coli* populations or the supplement SAMe.

f. Other enzyme deficiencies would need to be addressed with nutrition. Consider other remedies based on symptom presentation of the particular enzyme or vitamin deficiency.

g. Lactic acidosis: Deficiency of the enzyme lactate dehydrogenase, needed to metabolize lactic acid to lactate in the body, leads to hyper acidity, low oxygen, and results in low ATP production in cellular mitochondria. ***Natrum phosphoricum*** is indicated. Consider ***Rhus toxicodendron*** for excess lactic acid in the muscles.

h. Deficiency of lactate dehydrogenase is different than a glyphosate driven excessive histamine response to lactic acid that is not converted to acetic acid by deficient lacto-fermenting bacteria populations. ***Histaminum*** could be indicated in this situation. Consider ***Apis***, or ***Carbolic acid*** also for excess histamine responses.

i. Lactic acidosis from low oxygen levels in the system contributes to defective metabolism of the protein histamine. To address low oxygen levels consider ***Carbo vegetabilis***, ***Oxygenium***, ***Germanium***, ***Ferrum,*** or ***Sulphur*** based remedies including the cell salts. Low oxygen levels from prolonged fevers can drive lactic acidosis which forces septic conditions. Consider ***Ferrum phosphoricum***, ***Baptisia***, ***Pyrogenium***, ***Carbo vegetabilis***, or ***Lachesis*** to address fevers becoming septic or never been well since prolonged fevers. Lactic acidosis in this situation can be fatal if it is not urgently tended to.

IV. Collagen Issues:

Calcarea fluorica (Weak and overstretched ligaments), ***Calcarea sulphurica*** (deficient formation of collagen and lax fibers), ***Calcarea phosphorica***, (weak ligaments), ***Kali sulphuricum*** (formation of collagen), ***Natrum sulphuricum*** (stiff and brittle collagen), ***Causticum*** (contractures or paralysis), ***Graphites*** (excessive scar formation, knotting of collagen), ***Lachnanthes*** (stiffness, contractures and torticollis), ***Ledum*** (affinity to white fibrous tissue), ***Ruta*** (torn ligaments, stiffness, or contractures (from activation of mAChRs)), ***Silicea*** (weak structure, cannot stand erect), ***Thyroidinum*** (excess T4 weakens collagen). These remedies relate with fascia strength, contraction or relaxation, excessive production/ deterioration, in both tendons and ligaments. Copper is necessary for healthy collagen formation: consider ***Cuprum*** also in neurologic spasms and contractures due to activation of GPCRs. Prescribe based on symptoms: deformities, excessive scar formation, weak spine etc. Glyphosate renders a kind of contraction in the fascia when stimulated by the allergic response (histamine driven mast cell activation and degranulation) generated by foods high in glyphosate: torticollis, subluxations, and scoliosis are all within its realm of action. As Glyphosate's main influence is on the glycine needed in collagen formation and mast cell activation disease, ***Glyphosate*** may cure.

V. Liver and Metabolic Issues:

The liver governs protein metabolism, blood clotting, sugar and fat metabolism, bile production, and detoxification processes. All of which are affected by glyphosate. One of the main functions of the liver is liberation of nitrogen through the metabolism of protein and purines. The breakdown of proteins follows this course: Albumen → peptones → polypeptides → amino acids. This process is facilitated by enzymes. Amino acids are then chosen for reconstitution or passed through to → ammonia → ammonia carbonate, and eventually → urea to be released in the urine.

a. Remedies made from the various stages of this metabolic process will help when the system is stuck at that stage. Consider: ***Sulphur*** and sulfur-based remedies. ***Ammonium muriaticum***, ***Ammonium carbonicum***, ***Urea***, and other carbon or nitrogen based remedies such as ***Nitric acid***, ***Argentum nitricum***, ***Carbolic acid***, etc., to facilitate this pathway. Symptoms will demonstrate where the process is incomplete. E.g. ammoniacal smell of the perspiration or breath means that the enzymes needed to transform ammonia to urea are lacking.

b. **Phosphorus**: Quintessential for many liver functions. ***Phosphorus*** works on blood function (clotting and removal of damaged blood cells), bile and bile salt production, and fat metabolism. It works on the pancreas and sugar function with regards to insulin production and cellular absorption. Acts on strength of bones (with calcitonin), emulsification of fats, blood vessel strength, the parenchymal tissues, and nerve transmission. Uremia, hypoglycemia, hyperglycemia, diabetes, jaundice, blood clotting disorders, vomiting, and diarrhea.

c. **Nitrogen liberation from protein and purine metabolism**: Uremic acidosis, uric acid going towards gout, excessive blood clotting, increased sedimentation rates blood cells: nitrogenous remedies for any issues with nitrogen metabolism, tendency toward blood clotting issues, educations, hives, urticaria, gout etc. Embittered, resentful, angered, and vindictive feelings. Select remedies based on symptom expression: ***Nitric acid***, ***Ammonium*** salts, ***Apis, Benzoic acid, Berberis, Calcarea carbonica, Carbolic acid, China, Graphites, Lactic acid, Lycopodium, Sulphur, Sulphuric acid, Urea, Uric acid, Urtica urens***. Snake remedies. This is Stinging nettles' (***Urtica urens***) message to us:

> 'Pay attention, close your eyes, and become aware of the sun on your skin, and the breeze tickling your temples, and the rich scent of the earth, and the chuckle of the stream. Feel the complex and satisfying nourishment available to you where I live. And know that this is what I am: this complex nourishment of sun, wind, soil and water, transformed by my attention and my care, transformed into food for you, into milk for you.'[cxliv]

Stinging nettle, a weed killed by glyphosate, has the potential to treat many of the conditions created by glyphosate. And though not explicitly stated here, implicitly indicates its effect on Rhodopsin-like receptors, clear cognition, and experience of the natural world. ***Urtica urens*** addresses reduction in system wide inflammation, cerebral inflammation, lowers histamine, reduces neuro-toxicity of glutamate in the brain, reduces blood ammonia levels, and converts uric acid to urea increasing urine quality and output.

d. **Lithaemic acidosis**: Hyper elevated levels of uric acid in the blood, hives, joint inflammation.

Generalities; CONSTITUTION; lithaemic, acidosis, etc.: ant-c., aran., arn., berb., bry., calc., caust., chin., cocain., dulc., form., guai., kali-c., kalm., led., lith-c., lyc., med., mez., nat-s., rhod., rhus-t., sars., *sep.*, sulph., **Thuja**, ter.

e. **Ammonia from glutamate**: Magnesium dependent glutamine synthetase is utilized to make L-glutamine from potentially toxic glutamate. Its role depends on tissue localization: in the brain, it regulates the levels of ammonia and converts neurotoxic glutamate (calcium channel issues, hyperactivity, cerebral inflammation, schizophrenia) to harmless glutamine, whereas in the liver, it is one of the enzymes responsible for the metabolism of ammonia to urea (inability to do so makes hives, eczema, or gout). Consider: ***Belladonna*** (cerebral inflammation), ***Calcarea carbonica*** (calcium channels), ***Glonoinum*** (excess nitrogen in the brain), or ***Urea***, ***Uric acid***, or ***Urtica urens*** for hives, eczema, or gout, based on symptoms.

f. **Sulfate issues (sulfate depletion, methylation, and glutathione)**: ***Sulphur***, ***Sulphuric acid***, ***Antimonium crudum***, ***Allium cepa***, ***Chamomilla***, ***Lycopodium***, ***Carbolic acid***. (all remedies are high in sulfur) leading to skin issues, eczema, food sensitivities, immune system function, and protein metabolism issues. Consider these to be supportive remedies for those with MTHFR gene mutations.

g. **Other liver remedies*****:*** ***Bryonia*** in bile stagnation, pain on the right side. ***Colocynthis*** for colon spasms: must bend double. ***Chelidonium***: to pull bile, pain under the right shoulder blade. ***Aurum*** in fatty liver, depression, suicidal, hopelessness. ***Phosphorus*** for blood function, liver and bile, kidneys, bleeding, white stools, thirst, sugar metabolism issues ***Arsenicum;*** in metabolic allergic reactions, asthma, and anaphylaxis. ***Sulphur***, ***Lycopodium***, or ***Phosphorus*** or other remedy salts with ***Phosphorus*** also help the liver drain, address skin issues, and metabolic processes. ***Cholesterin*** to pull bile and lower cholesterol levels: low potency daily. ***Nux vomica*** to help detox drugs or food that the liver is insufficient in doing so.

Triticum monococcum (See 12. **Modern Wheat Vs Einkorn)** is a psoric remedy for all digestive issues, insufficient bile acids, conversion of bile acids to bile salts, elevated blood serum cholesterol, gallstones, bloating, diarrhea, constipation, blood sugar dysregulation, excessive urination, diabetes, infertility, and miscarriages. Einkorn wheat is rich in cobalamin (B12) and folate (B9) necessary for healthy fetal development. Most importantly ***Triticum monococcum*** is for treating the psoric feeling of lack, and fear for survival that drives the insatiable desire to steel the bounty of earth for profit. ***Triticum monococcum*** will help pull the bile, normalize blood sugar levels, and satiate any feelings of lack. It will help to normalize hormonal levels, ovulation and menstruation and bring us back in balance with the flow of the Mother Earth. If you find that eating Einkorn produces bloating or histamine reactions, consider ***Polio*** to close the tight junctions in the intestine. Herbal tinctures and nutritional support for the liver may also offer assistance in supporting healthy liver function. See my book **Homeopathic Therapeutics of the Liver and Biliary Ducts ~ The Amazing Liver: Interfacing Nature with Spirit** for more info. This book will help you address the various functions of the liver that may be disrupted by glyphosate toxicity.

VI. Kidney Issues:

a. Main remedies to think of to strengthen kidneys are ***Calcarea carbonica*** (calcium, kidney stones), ***Cannabis sativa***, ***Germanium***, ***Phosphorus***, ***Solidago***, ***Sarsaparilla***, ***Lycopodium***, ***Berberis***. Nettle tea, alfalfa tea, and barberry tincture.

b. **Nephrolithiasis – kidney stones**: A result of difficulty in metabolizing cysteine, oxalate and uric acid. Excess uric acid leads to excess phosphate in the blood which pulls calcium from the bones. Elevated homocysteine combined with phosphate calcifies leached calcium in the kidneys making kidney stones.

Urinary, KIDNEYS, Calculi: alum., ambr., **Ant-c.**, arn., berb., **Calc.**, calc-p., calc-r., **Cann-s.**, *canth.*, chin., lach., **LYC.**, nat-m., *nit-ac.*, *nux-m.*, **Nux-v.**, *petr.*, **Phos.**, **Ruta**, **SARS.**, **Sep.**, **Sil.**, *sulph.*, thuj., **Zinc.**

c. **Interstitial nephritis**: Inflammation of the tissues surrounding the tubules This may also be complicated by heavy metal toxicity.

Urinary; KIDNEYS; Inflammation: alum., **Bell.**, **Cann-s.**, **Canth.**, colch., hell., hep., kali-bi., *lyc.*, *merc.*, **MERC-C.**, **Nux-v.**, **PULS.**, sars.

d. **Kidney failure: *Digitalis*, *Pelias*, *Lachesis*, *Opium*, *Serum anguillae***, and more.
e. **Hypertension**: There are too many remedies to list here however I do want to point out that vasopressin and the hypothalamic-pituitary-adrenal axis and regulate blood pressure. The hormone remedies ***Posterior Pituitrin*** 30C, ***Vasopressin***, ***Adrenocorticotropic hormone (ACTH)*** 200C, ***Adrenal medulla/cortex*** 30C, in that order, may be needed in sequence to help organize healthy hormonal regulation. As per the table facing.

To normalize hypothalamic-pituitary-adrenal axis with hypertension.		
When	***Remedy***	Potency
Monday	***Pituitrin posterium***	30C
Tuesday	***Vasopressin***	200C
Wednesday	***Adrenal medulla/cortex***	30C
Pick a day	Give constitutional remedy	Best potency
Repeat cycle the following week and determine which gland or hormone is most affected based on which remedy lead to most improvement. Intercurrent constitutional remedy with the indicated sarcode.		

VII. Neurotransmitters, Acetylcholine, and GPCR Sites:

These are dependent on tryptophan and phenylalanine synthesis, the precursors, serotonin, glutamate, GABA, dopamine, and melatonin: the synthesis of which are all disrupted by glyphosate toxicity. Remedies for depression, flat affect, increased pain, deficient learning or memory, hyperactivity, insomnia (from lack of melatonin or adenosine receptor activation), suicidal ideation, schizophrenia, anxiety, and neurosis, are all signs of neurotransmitter imbalance and/or calcium channel or GPCR site dysfunction. Based on symptom expression there are several well-suited remedies that correspond to the specific receptor sites affected by glyphosate. Ligand gated Na^+, K^+, and Ca_2^+ channel and G-protein coupled receptors sites (GPCR): ACh receptor sites (nAChRs and mAChRs); Adenosine receptors (A1, A2a, A2b, A3); Serotonin receptors (5-HT); tryptamine or trace amine-associated receptors (TAAR); Glutamate receptor sites (NMDA receptors, AMPA receptors, delta receptors; kainite receptors) and other glycine dependent receptors.

Look for remedies based on mental and emotional states. Accordingly, these receptor sites will begin to work more effectively. Address biome and gut lining issues to correct neurotransmitter production. For those individuals on psycho-active prescription medication for anxiety, depression, hallucinations, etc. monitor care and withdrawal processes accordingly.

Generalities; CONSTITUTION; neuropathic: agar., ambr., arg-n., asaf., asar., aur., bell., cast., caust., cham., cimic., cina, cocc., coff., croc., **Ign.**, iod., kali-bi., kali-p., led., lil-t., mag-m., mag-p., mosch., **Nux-v.**, ph-ac., phos., pic-ac., puls., sel., sil., valer., zinc.

a. **Serotonin deficiency**: *Bifidobacteria* supplementation for tryptophan. Look to addressing the biome to address mental and emotional states. Take the case for constitutional prescribing and step-wise repair of gut, eliminatory processes, and mental states. Serotonin receptors (5-HT sites) are responsive to CBD oils and tryptamine sources (psychedelic plant alkaloids). CBD also releases the suppression of the immune system by temporarily deactivating the adenosine receptor sites. Aluminum detoxification also frees functionality of serotonin receptors

b. **For insomnia** first address the biome and its production of melatonin and serotonin. Then look at activated A2b adenosine receptor sites (see ***Carcinosin*** and subsequent reduced dopamine levels. Finally, if needed, treat hyperthyroid conditions. Consider a pattern like this:
    1. ***Candida*** and ***Natrum phosphoricum*** (plus probiotics) for 4 weeks (biome) followed by
    2. several repetitions of the sequence of ***Carcinosin*** and ***Glandular fever*** nosode, followed by the EBV specific remedy, based on symptoms of the previously experienced disease state (e.g. ***Phytolacca***, ***Phosphoric acid***, etc.). This series addresses the suppressed immune system and coinfection with EBV.
    3. Then ***Thyroidinum*** to support thyroid function.
    4. Treat based on the state with remedies that have affinities to these symptom presentations.

c. ***Calcarea carbonica*** for calcium channels in the brain and neurotransmitter functionality.

d. ***Natrum muriaticum*** for sodium, chlorine, and glutamate/GABA concentrations. As Na^+ and Cl^- open the receptor site gates for glutamate and GABA respectively.

e. **Ligand gated receptors (GPCRs)**: dependent upon minerals for their functioning. Copper (***Cuprum***), Zinc (***Zincum***), ***Brass***, and others.

f. **All conditions relating to reduced acetylcholinesterase(AChE)** activity leading to activation of the acetylcholine receptor sites. Glyphosate, organophosphorus, or carbamate insecticide poisonings are associated with reduced AChE activity. Atropine, hyoscyamine, and scopolamine are indicated for the management of poisoning by organophosphorus nerve agents (glyphosate is considered and organophosphorus nerve agent). These alkaloids are antagonists to both the nicotinic (NAChRs) and muscarinic (mAChRs) receptor sites (muscles, lungs, heart, salivation, perspiration etc.) that remain active under the influence of excess ACh. Consider ***Belladonna,***

Stramonium, ***Hyoscyamus*** as remedies with various concentrations of each alkaloid, or snake venoms like the black Mamba (***Dendroaspis polylepis***). ***Tabacum*** may be indicated in excessive activation of the nAChR sites of the vagus, sympathetic, cerebro-spinal nerves and heart. The alkaloids Muscarine (***Agaricus muscacrius*** (*Amanita muscacria*)), Physostigmine (***Physostigma***) or Pilocarpine (***Jaborandi***) both inhibit AChE activity in crude form at the mAChRs and may be indicated in paralysis, perspiration, salivation, pupil accommodation, etc. Also consider remedies indicated for *cholera* or *clostridial* neuro-toxic activation of ACh receptors: ***Ledum*** and ***Hypericum***, etc. *Tetanus* toxin blocks the release of ACh at the central nervous system cholinergic synapse causing spastic paralysis. ***Botulinum*** for blocked nAChRs at the peripheral synapse (where the nerve ending meets the muscle) causing flaccid paralysis. ***Clostridium difficile*** for intestinal pain. ***Curare***: paralysis of the lungs. ***Lathyrus sativus*** (paralysis of the lower limbs) and ***Physostigma*** (suffocation by paralysis of the lungs): both relate with polio toxin in the nervous system. Strychnine, from ***Nux vomica***, ***Ignatia***, or ***Gelsemium*** for paralysis or constriction of their respective organs of affinity.

g. **For excess adenosine** (activated adenosine receptor sites) induced lack of dopamine (insomnia and excessive wakefulness). The purines theobromine (chocolate) and caffeine (coffee) are antagonists to the adenosine receptors that are activated by glyphosate. Consider ***Chocolate*** or ***Coffea*** for excessive wakefulness. Also, ***Carcinosin*** as this remedy deactivates these sites. CBD oil and Cannabis related products also deactivate these sites by occupying them instead of the adenosine. While this action facilitates the release of the activation induced by these sites continued dosing of crude CBD oil is necessary to maintain the effect. See X. **Immune System** - a. **Histamine**, below for the effects of histamine and the adenosine receptors.

h. **Adenosine and acetylcholine (ACh)** together have, to a greater or lesser extent, an action on the adenosine receptor sites and the cholinergic signaling of the vagus nerve. Hydrocyanic acid activates adenosine receptor sites resulting in bronchospasm and cardiac relaxation. This combined action results in varying degrees of bronchospasm, cardiac arrest or relaxation, and/or, spasms/convulsions, or vomiting/diarrhea based on the food that is consumed or the mental or emotional state of the individual. Remember the vagus nerve, the "love" nerve, is regulated by acetylcholine. Constriction of the free flow of love, the energy from the unified field, can lead to a myriad of physical, mental, and emotional symptoms centered in the throat, heart, lungs, and alimentary track.

The Rosaceae family are a group of plants that produce edible fruit. These plants and fruits have relative concentrations of hydrocyanic acid, adenosine receptor site agonists, and cholinergic signaling agents. Acetylcholine is made from acetic acid and choline. Acetic acid is necessary for digestion of fatty acids, to regulate pH, and to reduce lactic acid. Anticholinergics are parasympatholytic agents that allow for the relaxation of the parasympathetic nervous system and vagus nerve, allowing the free flow feeling of love. These foods can act as anticholinergics or in individuals with food sensitivities can initiate allergic responses. In potency, as remedies, they can cure these same responses.

Some refer to these fruits as the 'nectar of the Gods:' they are fragrant, sweat, and juicy, and they house within them nutrients that satiate our need for love: that divine connection to benevolence of the universe that defines our Creation. They also have the capacity to heal deep disturbances in various physical manifestations and faulty understandings of love in relationship to another person. Two people can only love each other the amount they can love themselves and the degree to which each independently is conscious of, and connected to, the unified field.

Remedies are made from either the fruit itself or parts of the plant that grows the fruit. Not all members of the Rosaceae family have been made into remedies nor do we have the complete symptomatology of them all. Remedies are listed in accordance to Jan Scholten's schema if he had them cataloged.[cxlv] Some have limited referenceable physical or emotional symptoms.

Hydrocyanic acid: The most lethal poison known to man, this gas has been used in the ultimate form of lovelessness: extermination, as in Zyklon-B of the holocaust gas chambers. Convulsions, paralysis, constriction, suffocation, turning blue. Jaws clenched, rigid spasm, froths at the mouth.

Almond (***Amygdalus amara aqua***): Opisthotonos, violent convulsions, oppression of the chest, suffocative attacks, skin blue. Sleep inducing. Excessively brilliant eyes, sardonic laughter, joyful countenance.

Apple (***Malus pumila***): Beginning of love, should I continue in love? Is this the partner for me? Constriction of the throat.

Crab apple (***Malus pumila***): Delusion he's dirty, everything, food, himself. Delusion she is abused, molested, victim, being soiled or abased.

Blackthorn (***Prunus spinosa***): Oppression of chest, anxious respiration, and sharp, shooting neuralgias. The relationship is hard, they have to keep going but they are never satisfied.

Quince (***Cydonia vulgaris***): They have the delusion that their relationship is almost fulfilling, almost complete, but it still requires some minor adaptations, correction, or approval. Digestive ailments after deadly poisons, diarrhea, or dysentery. Repairs arterial plaques and lowers 'bad' cholesterol. It covers a wide range of pharmacological activities like cardiovascular, hypoglycemic, nephron-, hepato-, and UV-protective, aphrodisiac, antioxidant, anti-allergic, anti-atherosclerotic, antimicrobial, antibacterial, antifungal, antihypertensive, hypolipidemic, diuretic, antidiarrheal, antidepressant, antispasmodic, and anti-inflammatory effects.

Damas rose (***Rosa damascena***): Love is idealized in its most romantic form, as in the time of the troubadours, the medieval ideal of love, a love that will never come into form because it is too ideal and too idealized. Hay fever and allergies. Rosehip tea will lower adenosine levels, provide vitamin C, and reduce allergies.

Hawthorn (***Crataegus***): Rapid pulse, difficult respiration, and weak heart. Air hunger and high blood pressure. Pain in the heart and left arm. Trying to control the circumstances or the partner.

Blackberry (***Rubus fruiticosus***): The relationship is unfulfilling. They feel that they do not receive much love, although they themselves give too much. Heart palpitations.

Strawberry (***Fragaria vesca***): Anaphylaxis, swollen tongue and throat, faintness, choking, suffocation, and stroke. They know that the relationship is in fact over, but they keep waiting for their lover to come back one day, recognizing that the relationship had been true love.

Cherry laurel (***Laurocerasus***): Asphyxia, blueness, suffocation, gasps for air and clutches the heart. Epilepsy and clonic spasms with paralytic weakness. Fear and anxiety about imaginary evils. They have the delusion that no one loves them and that no one can love them. They think that they have lost all the love there is and are not lovable at all, so they don't even try to find love.

Peach (***Amygdalus persica***): Activation of the muscarinic acetylcholine receptors (mAChRs) resulting in vomiting and diarrhea. A good remedy for morning sickness.

Chokecherry (***Prunus virginiana***): Action on the heart with intermittent and deficient impulse. Wheezing and whistling in lungs.

Mountain ash (***Pyrus americanus***): Constriction of the lungs, spasm of the heart. As if the heart had stopped beating. Chilly. Sad but cannot cry. Feels clairvoyant: understands people's motives, gets out of her body walks around and returns.

Other remedies in acute conditions: ***Aconite***, ***Hydrobromic acid***, ***Mephitis***, ***Spongia***.

VIII. DNA and RNA:

Nearly twenty years ago, the idea that homeopathic remedies could interact with the summation of all the messenger RNA molecules began to be formerly tackled. RNA is the messenger of the DNA encrypted genes of an organism and induces the manifestation of these genes. Subsequently, various investigations have established that homeopathic therapies do have the ability to upsurge the manifestation of many genes. We now call this epigenetics. Two remedies, ***Cundurango*** and ***Hydrastis canadensis*** have the capability to re-organize the manifestation of more than a hundred genes. Both remedies are thought of in end stage cancer.

Carcinosin, Carcinosin co., Carcinosin T58 are of vital importance to ensure healthy DNA and RNA replication, gene editing, and cellular integrity. Dose weekly.

All constitutional remedies do have the ability to affect epigenetics: They can affect the outcome of the DNA coded plan by addressing the functionality of RNA editing enzymes. It is logical that the mineral remedies that create the basic life forms, ***Oxygenium***, ***Carbon***, ***Nitrogen***, and ***Hydrogen***, or any mineral remedies from these combined base elements would constitutionally, greatly affect the outcome of any changes in formation of the nucleotides DNA and RNA (composed of O-C-N-H). Additionally, the phosphate group attached to the ribose or deoxyribose back bone of RNA or DNA, respectively, implicate ***Phosphorus*** as a major player in DNA replication and transcription. ***Sulphur*** and ***Silicea*** are fundamental to all living organisms, therefore provide a foundation of constitutional support.

Deoxyribonucleic acid (DNA) remedy influences gene expression. The ability of the message to manifest in life. ***DNA*** is indicated in Psoric constitutions for allergic symptoms, insomnia, hyperthyroidism, gene mutations, or cancer. On the mental sphere: difficulty assembling thoughts, loosing track of what she was to do, impossible to work, physical and mental backwardness, lack of willpower to finish tasks, mania, and irritability. Feels broken and does not know his purpose. *Note on source. Most pharmacies carry only fish ***DNA***. Select pharmacies carry human ***DNA***. For humans it would be better to go with human ***DNA***.

Ribonucleic acid (RNA) remedy, the messenger of the code. Covers psoric, cancer and tubercular constitutions. Presenting symptoms are hunger for sugar, rapid loss of weight, tired, sleepy, and hungry, as if living on one's nerves. Unable to complete a task, inability for intention to come to fruition. Lost communication, getting lost on the street. Messages not going through.

IX. Endocrine System:

The hypothalamic-pituitary-adrenal and -thyroid axes governs the functioning and feedback loops of hormones and glands in the endocrine system. These axes are disrupted by glyphosate on multiple levels leading to systemic endocrine issues. The living biome is the main director of catecholamine production (sex hormones) and their influence within the endocrine system: many endocrine functions will normalize once the biome is re-established. Start treatment with the biome then intercurrent specific glandular sarcodes with constitutional remedies depending on symptoms and targeted glandular issues. Suggested protocols are listed after the table on the next page.

Gland-Hormone	Purpose	Target Gland	Sarcodes	Related remedies
Anterior pituitary gland releases			***Anterior pituitrin*** (Most sarcodes are sourced from sheep or cow glands)	
Growth hormone (GH)	Growth		***HGH***	***Carcinosin***
Human chorionic gonadotropin	Growth of fetus and suppression of mother's immune system		***HCG***	
Thyroid stimulating hormone (TSH)	Synthesis and secretion of thyroid hormones. The parathyroid gland regulates calcium and calcitonin levels.	Thyroid gland. Para-thyroid.	***Thyroidinum, Para-thyroidinum.***	***Iodatum, Kali iodatum, Ferrum iodatum, Tuberculinum, Calcarea carbonica***
Adreno-cortico-tropic hormone (ACTH)	Stimulation of the synthesis and secretion of androgen and aldosterone,	Adrenal Medulla/ Cortex	***Adreno-corticotropic hormone (ACTH),***	Remedies for fight or flight responses,

			Adrenal medulla/cortex Adrenaline (from the medulla), ***Cortisone acetate*** (from the cortex).	Vagus nerve, or Acetylcholine antagonists.
Follicle stimulating hormone (FSH)	Growth and release of the ovarian follicles. Stimulation of testes and release of sperm.	Ovarian follicles. Testicular follicles.	***Oophorinum***, ***Foliculinum***, ***Orchitinum***.	Remedies for infertility ***Sepia***, ***Thuja***, ***Onchorinus*** (Salmon).
Luteinizing hormone (LH)	Synthesis of testosterone, stimulates ovulation, formation of the corpus luteum and the conversion of androgen to estrogen and progesterone.	Ovarian follicles. Testicular follicles.	***Testosterone, Estrogen, Progesterone.***	
Prolactin	Secretion of milk and the growth of mammary glands.		***Prolactin***	***Conium***, ***Phytolacca***, ***Lac*** remedies (***Lac Caninum***).
Gland-Hormone	Purpose	Target Gland	Sarcodes	Related remedies
Posterior pituitary gland releases:			***Pituitrin posterium***	
Vasopressin	Regulates the retention of water and blood pressure.	Kidneys	***Vasopressin***	Remedies for Hypertension: ***Natrum*** salts, ***Kali*** salts

Oxytocin	Production and release of milk, induces uterine contractions, parturition and orgasm.	Breasts, cervix, and uterus.	***Oxytocin***	Remedies for labor: failure to progress.

a. **Catecholamine dysregulation**: Hormones produced by the adrenal glands, which sit on top of the kidneys: dopamine, epinephrine (adrenaline), and norepinephrine. These are made from a tyrosine base, which is derived from dietary sources as well as being synthesized from phenylalanine. Phenylalanine is produced in bacteria via the shikimate-acid pathway.

b. **Thyroid function**: ***Anterior pituitrin***, ***Thyroidinum***, ***Parathyroidinum***, and other remedies as listed above. Thyroid driven birth defects cannot be cured with homeopathy. Intercurrent with appropriate remedies. Consider ***Calcarea carbonica*** for calcitonin deficiency and hypothyroidism. See X. **Immune System** for clearing Epstein-Barr virus (EBV) driven thyroiditis. ***Tuberculinum***, ***Iodine***, or ***Ferrum*** salts for hyperthyroidism as the enzyme for thyroxine (T4) to Triiodothyronine (T3) conversion is heme-dependent.

c. **Adrenal gland – Endocrine driven elevated histamine**: ***Anterior pituitrin*** or ***Cortisone acetate*** if the condition appears to be endocrine related. ***Histaminum*** 200C weekly also. ***Cortisone acetate*** especially if there has been a history of steroid usage to suppress inflammation. Suggested dosage 9C for several weeks. Or use the remedies in sequence to repair adrenal dysfunction (one dose of one remedy per day; repeat cycle 2-3 times). Use this sequence to determine which gland or hormone is not responsive in the feed-back loop by the response to the remedy in the person.\

d. **Adrenal gland – Elevated cortisol**: Some say low potencies stimulate response and high potencies suppress response. In the following chart we are asking the gland to release the correct amount of hormone with the 30C, and the hormones released to be held in check with the 200C. In this case of hyper-elevated release of cortisone, we would want to stimulate the glands and suppress the release of excess ACTH and cortisol.

To normalize the hypothalamic-pituitary-adrenal axis in adrenal over drive.		
Time	***Remedy***	Potency
Day 1	***Anterior pituitrin***	30C
Day 2	***Adrenocorticotropic hormone (ACTH)***	200C
Day 3	***Adrenal medulla/cortex***	30C
Day 4	***Cortisone acetate***	200C
Day 5	***Adrenaline***	200C
Repeat cycle then determine which gland or hormone is most affected by most improvement and intercurrent constitutional remedy with indicated sarcode.		

e. **Sex hormone balance and infertility**: ***Oophorinum***, ***Foliculinum***, ***Anterior pituitrin***, ***Adrenal medulla/cortex***, ***Testosterone***. Be sure to address vaginal pH balance. While the vagina needs an acidic environment, if it is too acidic the sperm will die: ***Natrum phosphoricum*** will help to moderate system pH.

f. **Gonad stimulation in the female**: To regulate the hormonal cycle give ***Foliculinum*** 200C before menses day 24, and ***Oophorinum*** 30C day 12. If Cycle is coming every three weeks give ***Oophorinum*** on day 10 for a few cycles, then stretch out to day 12-14. In cases of breakthrough or prolonged bleeding or delayed menstruation give ***Thlaspi*** 200C on day 5 of bleeding to stop the bleeding and mother tincture, *Shepard's purse,* on day 26 to bring on the menses. Check which ovary is releasing in alternating lengths of monthly cycles and treat with associated remedies: ***Apis*** for right-sided-cysts, ***Lachesis*** for left-sided etc.

   I am unclear if homeopathy can help if ovarian cycle relationships have been altered in perinatal development. If glyphosate driven hormonal disturbances are further confounded by the HPV vaccine, or previous synthetic hormonal use (birth control, infertility drugs, hormone augmented childbirth, or menopausal issues), work to address these issues with appropriate vaccine or synthetic hormone tautopathic detoxification first.

To normalize the female ovarian cycle		
Time	***Remedy***	Potency
Day 12-14 depending on length of cycle.	***Oophorinum***	30C
Day 24.	***Foliculinum***	200C
As needed.	***Constitutional remedy***	30C
Each sat or Mon-Fri.	***Thuja*** in cases of polycystic ovaries.	200C or 30C
Repeat cycle monthly until ovulation is consistent and cycle has normalized.		

g. **Gonad stimulation in the male**:

To support male sterility/sperm defects		
Time	***Remedy***	Potency
Each Sat.	***Testosterone***	30C
Ass needed: Weekly.	Constitutional remedy	200C
Each Sunday or Mon-Fri.	Sperm motility issues consider ***Calcarea carbonica*** for calcitonin issues), ***Manganum*** (for nAChRs issues)	30C
Repeat cycle monthly until ovaries are consonantly releasing and cycle has normalized.		

h. **Neonatal development**: ***Tuberculinum*** - ***Anterior pituitrin*** - ***Thyroidinum***, ***Human chorionic gonadotropin (HCG)*** deficiency leads to excess adrenaline which equals under developed cerebral cortex. ***Tuberculinum*** has an affinity to the pituitary gland and its control of the endocrine system. Tuberculosis will calcify the functionality of the gland. The nosode would decalcify its function. Multiple doses may be necessary over a long period of time.

i. **Blood pressure**: ***Pituitrin posterium*** then ***Vasopressin:*** excessive urination, and constipation. Pituitary dysfunction: ***Pituitrin posterium***. Failure to progress in labor, ailments from parturition. For hypertension from induced labor add ***Pitocin*** 200C in this cycle.

To normalize the hypothalamic-pituitary-adrenal axis in adrenal over drive.		
Time	***Remedy***	Potency
Day 1	***Pituitrin posterium***	30C
Day 2	***Vasopressin***	200C
Day 3	***Adrenal medulla/cortex***	30C
Day 4	Constitutional remedy	200C
Repeat cycle weekly then determine which gland or hormone is most affected by most improvement and intercurrent constitutional remedy with indicated sarcode.		

j. **cAMP pathway**: Calcitonin is the main driver for the G-protein coupled receptors involved in cyclic adenosine monophosphate pathways (cAMP). These pathways allow for a cascade of signaling processes that regulate the entire endocrine system. Calcium concentrations are regulated by adenosine receptor sites and the parathyroid gland. Consider ***Parathyroidinum*** or ***Calcarea carbonica*** to normalize calcitonin levels and cAMP signaling pathways. Eat oysters for calcium to supercharge the hormonal system, release acetylcholine, stimulate the vagus nerve, and increase the potential for orgasm.

X. Immune System:

The main target of glyphosate on the immune system is suppression through activation of the adenosine receptors and interference with purinergic signaling and editing of DNA replication and RNA transcription.

a. Histamine reactions are driven by several functions in relationship to glyphosate. Accordingly, different remedies may be needed to work different pathways.
    i. **Excess lactic acid driven elevated histamine**: Allergic responses to lacto-fermenting bacteria: ***Lacticum acidum*** and ***Natrum phosphoricum*** for excess lactic acid. Intercurrent and use daily for several weeks. ***Histaminum***, ***Rheum***, ***Calcarea carbonica***, ***Natrum lacticum, Natrum muriaticum***, ***Apis***.
    ii. **Mast Cell Activation disease**, allergic asthma, anaphylaxis, or hives: a combined result of zinc dependent ADA deficiency and resultant excess adenosine, activating the adenosine receptor sites: A1, A2b, and A3, deficiency in histamine-N-methyltransferase, and/or elevated IgE antibody levels leads to a food driven excessive histamine response. In acute conditions ***Carcinosin*** is the first remedy to think of in that it pulls the adenosine off the receptor sites by releasing suppression of the immune system. Based on symptoms: ***Apis***, ***Arsenicum***, ***Adrenaline***, ***Carbolic acid***, ***Cortisone acetate***, ***Fragaria***, ***Histaminum, Homarus***, ***Lycopodium***, ***Ledum***, ***Natrum muriaticum***, ***Rhus toxicodendron***, ***Torula***, ***Vespa***, ***Zincum***.
    iii. Histamine can also be elevated by excess uric acid in the system from metabolic issues. Refer to V**. Liver and Metabolic Issues** for more info.

b. **Adenosine receptor site driven bronchospasm**: This is an emergency condition and will be attended with rapid heart rate. Main remedy is ***Carcinosin*** as it actively reduces adenosine levels. Dose ***Carcinosin*** 200C in water. Sip every ten minutes for thirty minutes, then once an hour until episode has passed. Caffeine and theobromine (Chocolate) are antagonists to these sites. These may be helpful in crude form in emergency conditions to counter act the spasm. ***Coffea*** or ***Chocolate*** in potency are interesting to consider. See VII. **Neurotransmitters, Acetylcholine, and GPCRs** for more on the interface of adenosine receptors, Adenosine deaminase (ADA) activity, and acetylcholine receptors.

c. Consider the role of acetylcholine, histamine and adenosine on the constriction of the lungs and think of the remedies that act as muscarinic receptor antagonists: ***Podophyllum***, ***Jaborandi***, ***Tabacum***, ***Curare***, and remedies in the Rosacea family.

d. **Co-infections with retroviruses**: The remedy of import here is ***Carcinosin*** and its ability to upregulate the immune system to keep these retroviruses in check. Also consider ***Zincum*** to activate adenosine deaminase (ADA) to release adenosine from the adenosine receptor sites or ***Cuprum*** to normalize copper concentrations. ***Cuprum***, ***Zincum***, or ***Brass*** (a combination of the two) should be given in lower potency (nutritional dosing, x potencies or 30C)) and nosodes given in higher potency (200C). You may need to set a course with the specific disease nosode, e.g. ***Glandular fever*** nosode (EBV), ***Herpes*** nosode, ***HIV*** nosode, ***Hepatitis B*** etc. Remember organ specific cancer nosodes. Consider ***Carcinosin co.*** or ***Carcinosin T58***, or ***Cuprum cum Carcinosin***. Other viruses can also be cleared in the following way.

To clear never been well since infective conditions, e.g. Epstein-Barr virus.		
Time	***Remedy***	Potency
Friday	***Carcinosin***	200C
Saturday	***Glandular fever*** or other viral nosode.	200C
Sunday	Main indicated remedy from first occurrence. Must be able to treat glandular fever (Epstein-Barr virus (EBV).	30C three times in one day
Rest until the next weekend or two weeks		
Friday	***Carcinosin***	200C three times in one day
Saturday	***Glandular fever*** or other viral nosode.	200C three times in one day
Sunday	Main indicated remedy from first occurrence.	30C three times in one day
Expect a fever and return of old symptoms. Repeat cycle in 1M if necessary. Allow two weeks to one month to rest between cycles.		

e. **Vaccine co-morbidity**: Please refer to CEASE Therapy to learn more about vaccine damage and its relation to ADD, ADHD, autism, cerebral inflammation and auto-immune disease. Certainly, glyphosate toxicity will add to the chronic inflammation from vaccine introduced RNA and Retroviruses.

It is suggested to do a multi-vaccine-clearing-protocol first to reduce the inflammation first, to resolve the immune system occupation stimulated by the injected viral or bacterial antigens. Follow with 16. **Glyphosate Clearing Protocol.**

Symptoms common to vaccine induced cerebral inflammation include: teeth grinding, laughing immoderately, biting, desire to escape or run away, hitting oneself or bystanders, jumping, throwing things. Sound and light sensitivity, sound of water, avoids eye contact. Nervous system is stuck in fight or flight, cannot learn, or over-active memory. Consider MMR vaccine clearing or ***Morbillinum*** in demyelization.
Consider ***Polio*** for tight junction issues. Or the following in any cases of vaccine induced cerebral inflammation (brain cry).

Consider these remedies: **mind; SHRIEKING,** screaming, shouting; brain cry (50): ***Aml-n.***, **APIS**, arn., ars., ***Art-v.***, bell., bor., **BRASS**, bry., calc., calc-hp., canth., ***Carb-ac.***, ***Cham.***, cic., ***Cina***, coff., crot-c., **CUPR.**, ***Cupr-acet.***, cupr-ar., cypr., dig., dpt, dulc., gels., ***Glon.***, ***Hell.***, ***Hyos.***, ign., iodof., ***Kali-br.***, ***Kali-i.***, lac-h., ***Lyc.***, merc., merc-c., merc-v., nux-m., per., phos., plb., ***Rhus-t.***, ***Sol-n.***, ***Solin.***, stram., sulph., syph., tub., verat-v., ***Zinc.***

More specifically look at the remedies relating to *Clostridia* species toxins and/or disease specific for suppressed exanthema, excess lactic acid, aluminum toxicity, mercury toxicity, insufficient fevers, excess glutamate/GABA deficiency, copper/zinc ratios and glyphosate driven cerebral inflammation.

Cancer*:* Cancer is an end stage disease. By the time an individual has cancer there may not be enough vital energy in the person to heal the cancer. However, all physical and nutritional detoxes, as introduced in this book, along with select remedies can substantially improve the health. ***Carcinosin*** is the main remedy, but then others based on symptoms and pathogenesis will be indicated. ***Carcinosin*** will release the adenosine suppression of the immune system. Check for latent retro, RNA, or herpes viruses being activated. Iron deficiency, heavy metal toxicity, poor oxygenation, poor diet, increased toxic load from ineffective colon elimination, suppressed emotions, grief, and anger all have the potential to develop into cancer. Cancer is about the under-differentiated person in an undifferentiated life. The cells regress to an undifferentiated state. We all have the potential for cancer within us. Improper use of our energy system and failure to maintain a healthy relationship with ourselves as creative individuals is the first step in moving towards cancer. Secondarily, maintaining interdependent rather than co-dependent relationships with other people, ensures the susceptibility to cancer be reduced.

Start with cleaning up the biome, and ensuring the liver and kidneys are eliminating property. Then address latent viruses occupying the immune system, adenosine receptor activation, and suppression of the immune system.

There are too many remedies to list here but consider ***Calcarea phosphorica*** in bone cancer and tendency to cancer, ***Thuja*** in hyperproliferation of cells, ***Phytolacca*** in extensive glandular involvement, ***Ceanothus*** in anemia and enlarged spleen, ***Hydrastis*** for gene mutations, ***Acetic acid*** in severe anemia and iron deficiency, and others.

---

cxlii Christine Stabell Benn. How vaccines train the immune system in ways no one expected. TEDxAarhus. https://www.youtube.com/watch?v=_d8PNlXHJ48.

cxliii Judy A. Mikovits, Vincent C. Lombardi, Max A. Pfost, Kathryn S. Hagen, Francis W. Ruscetti. Detection of an infectious retrovirus, XMRV, in blood cells of patients with chronic fatigue syndrome. Virulence. 2010. Sep-Oct; 1(5): 386–390. https://www.ncbi.nlm.nih.gov/pmc/articles/PMC3073172/.

cxliv Susan Weed. Wise woman Herbal: Healing Wise. Ash Tree Publishing. April 11, 2003.

cxlv Jan Scholten, Deborah Collins. Introduction to the Rosaceae family. December 2012. http://www.interhomeopathy.org/introduction-to-the-rosaceae-family.

16. Glyphosate Clearing Protocol

As per the schedule next page, use the ***Glyphosate*** homeopathic remedy in ascending potencies: 30C-10M, over an eight-week course. Each potency is to be taken. Two weeks at each potency, or one week per potency, or two-four weeks per potency, depending on the health of the individual. Match the potency duration to the amount and ability of the body to liberate glyphosate. All supplementation in the previous tables must be taken during this clearing protocol, most especially on the days when taking ***Glyphosate***. Potentized ***RoundUp*** can also be used in a similar course. You can do both during the same course: alternate Monday and Wednesday (***Glyphosate***) with Tuesday and Thursday (***RoundUp***) in the same week if necessary. The days off on the schedule are rest days.

This protocol may need to be repeated after six months or upon new exposure. As the body normally detoxes in layers, only the most peripheral glyphosate will be released the first time through. Stores of glyphosate in the collagen and liver may take years to be fully released. Re-exposure will cause the condition to relapse. Be sure to supplement nutrition Monday, Tuesday, and Wednesday. Incorporate other foods in these days and throughout the week.

1. In the a.m. before breakfast
    a. ***Glyphosate*** remedy at indicated potency
    b. Collagen supplement one scoop or six capsules
    c. Digestive enzymes
    d. Probiotics
    e. Fat soluble vitamin C
    f. Fresh squeezed grapefruit juice
2. P.m. with dinner
    a. Digestive enzymes
    b. Probiotics
    c. Fat soluble vitamin C
3. P.m. before bed. Mix with juice or apple cider vinegar
    a. Activated charcoal
    b. Bentonite clay
    c. Psyllium husks.

Follow this schedule to clear glyphosate. Repeat in few months along with nutritional support and detoxification.

Core supplementation during this phase: Collagen, Ascorbyl Palmitate, Digestive Enzymes, and Probiotics.			
		3 pellets a day per dose	Note reaction
Weeks 1 and 2	***Glyphosate*** 30C	Monday, Tuesday, and Wednesday	
	Intercurrent remedy		
Weeks 3 and 4	***Glyphosate*** 200C	Monday, Tuesday, and Wednesday	
	Intercurrent remedy		
Weeks 5 and 6	***Glyphosate*** 1M	Monday, Tuesday, and Wednesday	
	Intercurrent remedy		
Weeks 6 and 7	***Glyphosate*** 10M	Monday, Tuesday, and Wednesday	
Intercurrent on Saturdays, or other weekdays, with indicated remedies.		Consult your homeopath for indicated remedies.	

17. Clients in Practice

Since I became aware of my own toxicity from glyphosate, I have now realized how this has impacted some of my clients located in the Midwest. Particularly those children that live in rural communities adjacent to farmland and the famers who now have cancer, kidney disease, gout, or other demonstrations of toxicity. More recently, I am recognizing glyphosate toxicity in various city dwelling clients with the familiar gut dysbiosis and general malaise, headaches from wine, gluten intolerance, failure to heal, gastrointestinal irritability, and excessive histamine issues, mast cell activation disease, and *Candida*. These individuals are at various stages of the detox protocol.

1. **VW, 6-year-old girl**:

VW lives in Iowa. Her father is a farmer who sprays glyphosate on his crops. She came to me with vaccine induced allergic conditions, eczema, asthma, and some behavioral issues.

After 6-8 months of clearing the vaccines through homeopathic vaccine detox protocols her health was significantly improved. However, we reached a plateau in improvement. What remained were seasonal episodes of life-threatening asthmatic conditions. Her airways would constrict and go into bronchospasm with rapid respiration and heart rate after any extended exposure to non-air-conditioned air during the intense spraying seasons (spring and fall). She has responded well to ***Apis***, ***Arsenicum***, ***Histaminum***, and ***Carcinosin***.

The last episode was coupled with a cold that progressed into pneumonia. This resolved with ***Pneumococcinum*** and ***Kali bichromicum***, which cleared the mucus and pneumonia symptoms, followed by ***Carcinosin*** when all that remained was the bronchospasm. ***Carcinosin*** 200C, in water, sipped every ten minutes over a few hours, complctcly released the bronchospasm.

Comments: It is my understanding that it was an excess of adenosine activating the A1 and A2b receptor sites. ***Carcinosin*** actively blocks these sites thus reducing this purinergic signaling driven process.

2. **SM, Female aged 24:**

What follows is a narration of a young woman who grew up in Iowa. "My journey to health began 13 years ago at the age of 17. I started having trouble breathing, brain fog, muscle aches and tension, sensitivity to fragrances, and fatigue from all of that. Through the years I tried many different modalities, osteopathic manipulative medicine, chiropractic, GAPS, dietary measures, homeopathy, and others. Most helped in some degree and all have contributed to the healing process, but nothing cleared up the symptoms and gave me sustained healing.

"I liked homeopathy and knew it to be effective so after the homeopath I was working with retired I sought to find a new homeopath. I began working with Kate Birch. This time, along with working on my individual symptoms, I was also put on a **Glyphosate Clearing Protocol**. ***Lachnanthes*** covered the symptoms of my torticollis: contraction and twisting of the collagen in my spine. ***Glyphosate*** was given in ascending potencies along with the nutritional support discussed in this book.

"I was suffering from symptoms of anemia when I first started that cleared up very quickly with the correct remedy (***Ferrum phosphoricum***) and shortly after I began the **Glyphosate Clearing Protocol**. This clearing has quite literally changed my life. I began to see results very quickly, the brain fog by this point was not as prominent, but the muscle issues – tension, achiness, and then difficulty breathing – were all very much present. Once I started the glyphosate protocol things got better. The tension reduced, I was less sensitive to scents, the achiness began to abate, and I could breathe!

"A couple months later the symptoms began to return in a milder form, and I was able to repeat the glyphosate protocol to eradicate the symptoms. As I live in Iowa, in a farming area which is heavily sprayed with Roundup, again, after a couple months in the spring spraying season the precursors to another flare up begin to show themselves. This was corrected again with the removal of glyphosate from my system by repeating the homeopathic **Glyphosate Clearing Protocol.**

"My symptoms may return, in this age of environmental toxins and the constant desire to spray weed killer, it's impossible to avoid contact with glyphosate. The important thing is that I now have a way of combating it and restoring my body to balance and for that I am thankful."

Comments: In this case her system is mostly affected by glyphosate disruption of her gut biome and digestive process, iron absorption, and muscle tension caused by glyphosate in her collagen and fascia. Continued exposure will be an issue as she lives in the Midwest. ***Ferrum phosphoricum*** helped her body absorb iron and stimulated her body to make more red blood cells. ***Lachnanthes*** is a remedy for torticollis, a condition marked by twisting of the spine due to contraction of the collagen. Constitutionally, ***Silicea*** has maintained her health.

3. **HL, 4-year-old girl**:

At six months of age HL had extensive massive glyphosate exposure when her family moved to a new house in the farm land of Western Minnesota. The previous owners were conventional farmers and the water for the house pulls from a well on the land. Very shortly after moving into this house she started to develop hives, and welts which over the next weeks and months progressed to systemic urticaria and spread head to toe as a weeping dermatitis.

Over the years she has had bouts of urinous smelling skin, malnutrition, and failure to thrive because of her systemwide allergic response to nearly all food. She is small for her age and suffers from protein malnutrition because she cannot metabolize any proteins without an excessive histamine reaction. To ease the histamine reactions the mother has limited most protein sources. At four years of age she can now digest some meat, eggs, and salmon with daily intake of enzymes.

We started our homeopathic journey at six months of age with remedies based on symptoms. Several of the remedies helped for some amount of time, but none cured: ***Candida***, ***Lycopodium***, ***Urtica urens***, ***Apis***, ***Natrum muriaticum***, ***Antimonium crudum***, ***Histaminum***, ***Carcinosin***, ***Arsenicum***, ***Lithium carbonicum*** and ***Sulphur***. Each remedy was used in 30C or 200C potency over extended periods.

I am not sure if cure is possible for her because they live next door to other farmlands that are sprayed with glyphosate each season and her early exposure may have contaminated her DNA to an extent that she will continue to be enzyme deficient and cannot detox it. We had done the **Glyphosate Clearing Protocol**, which in the beginning improved her skin but, in the end, made it worse. This protocol was also done during the fall spraying season, so the aggravation may just have been from more exposure. In the last year we added ***Torula*** for the excessive histamine response to proteins. Follow up is due.

During spraying seasons HL's symptoms get worse. It was not until the fall of 2017 (at three years of age) that we realized this was glyphosate toxicity. This girl cries from the itching and burning in her skin. Remedies hold only for a short amount of time, and the **Glyphosate Clearing Protocol** initially helped by then aggravated her skin. We started on ***Cortisone acetate*** 200c to help down-regulate histamine production, ***Natrum phosphoricum*** 9x daily to address the excess reaction to lactic acid from enzyme deficiency of the conversion of lactic acid to acetic acid, and ***Lactic acid*** 200C weekly to help with that part of lactic acid metabolism. She takes enzymes daily, bentonite clay baths each night, and her diet is critically watched so as to limit allergenic foods.

Comments: Her biggest issue is continued exposure to glyphosate in the well water from their farm which includes run off from theirs and the neighboring farmlands. The effect on her has been a significant enzyme deficiency leading to in ability to digest proteins and purines, uric acid build up due to excess nitrogen, the inability to convert lactic acid to lactate, excessive histamine reaction from elevated lactic acid, *Candida* over growth, kidney inflammation, and dermatitis. I believe that glyphosate was incorporated into her DNA, and she is not coding for the enzymes correctly. For her, this toxicity has crippled her system and trying to navigate our way through to cure has been difficult.

The assistance of multiple practitioners with a variety of modalities are needed to support her.

Through the research required to write this book I understand HL's health/disease pattern more significantly and am working to hone prescriptions more accurately. Deduction of these conditions came through understanding the symptom presentations. Muscle testing and responses to foods and supplements have confirmed these findings. At this time the skin lesions have been reduced to her lower leg, inner thighs, wrists, and ankles. In time we are hoping to help her with the occasional systemic hives brought on by food or emotional dysregulation.

4. **JJ, 52-year-old woman. 10/3/18**:

"My name is Janan. I am 52 years of age, I am a Pastry Chef, and live in MN. My first food allergy began over six years ago with wheat/gluten intolerance, and then an intolerance to dairy five years ago when I started Pastry School. I had severe constipation alternating with severe diarrhea. I developed asthma around the same time and carried an inhaler for several years. I developed a burning throat immediately after eating and drinking. I decided to remove gluten and dairy from my diet five years ago even though my family physician refused to believe food was causing my health problems. Within a month, my asthma disappeared, and my digestion slightly improved. However, two years ago, I started developing high histamine reactions to almost all food. My energy was extremely low, some days I could barely get out of bed to eat breakfast. My digestion nearly halted. The only relief I could find was through several enemas a week. I reacted not only to food, but to everything in my environment – from EMF's in my home to simple odors at the grocery store, lighting, sound, and to negative people (I felt hurt and crushed emotionally). I was forced to close my cake business in order to care for myself.

"I continued to struggle with my failing health while searching for answers and received various medical tests from blood work to Genova Diagnostics Stool Profile, Meridian Valley Food Panel Analysis, Colonoscopy, hormone panel, Saliva/Cortisol analysis, SIBO test,

Tryptase test (excreted from mast cells in allergic responses), CT scan, Great Plains Organic Acids Test, Endoscopy, and even a psychological evaluation – all tests were 'normal' except for the Endoscopy which revealed high levels of CD117 mast cells. Even with a MCAS diagnosis, I could not find a cause for my health problems and continued to get sicker, developing burning mouth syndrome, oral allergy syndrome, acid reflux, severe constipation alternating with severe diarrhea, fatigue, low energy, foggy brain, weight loss, and emotionally becoming very reactive to negative people/situations (easily hurt by others).

I had experienced an interesting response to food/drink while vacationing in France for six weeks in April/May 2018. I was able to eat and drink anything I desired in France and returned to Minnesota in better health than when I left (good energy, good digestion, healthy skin, emotionally positive). Within two weeks of my return to the US, my health deteriorated to the original state.

"I received a homeopathic intake with Kate Birch on July 5, 2018. I began the **Glyphosate Clearing Protocol** on July 31, 2018 as directed with ***Natrum phosphoricum*** 9X daily, as well as ***Histaminum*** 30C; ***Conium*** 200C on Saturday and ***Cortisone acetate*** 200C on Sunday. I experienced dizziness for the first day of the protocol (***Glyphosate*** 30), as well as the beginning of Week 2, but this subsided thereafter. I did not notice any changes in my health during Week 1 through 4.

I met with Kate around week 4, and ***Conium*** was removed and a new digestive enzyme (Digest-a-Zyme) was added along with ***Aqua amniotica*** 30C (Thursday through Saturday). By week 5 (beginning of (***Glyphosate*** 1M) I felt significantly better – great energy, emotionally positive, regular bowel movements, weight gain, little fatigue. I continued to experience histamine reactions and burning tongue symptoms, along with acid reflux. I added Jovial Foods organic Einkorn wheat to my diet without a reaction.

"Since doing the eight-week glyphosate detox, I am feeling like a completely different person! My digestion is really good – I have regular normal bowel movements, and food seems to move through my system without trouble (no more weekly enemas!). My energy is positive and lasts through the day/evening. I no longer need daily naps. I am no longer reactive or hurt by people's comments. I can sense their negative energy, and either avoid them completely or put up a bubble and shield to avoid the effects of their energy. I can think clearly, and my memory is razor sharp! My histamine response is less, and I am able to eat an increased variety of foods. At week 9 and 10, I continue to notice improvement in my health. My tongue no longer burns which is remarkable, as it has burned daily for over two years! I am now thinking about re-opening my designer cake business using Einkorn wheat!"

Comments: In my assessment, the excessive exposure and consumption of wheat during pastry school was enough to completely disrupt the intestinal biome thereby reducing available trypsin to digest gluten and reduce myosin levels to the point of intestinal smooth muscle paralysis and gallbladder inactivity resulting in limited bile salts to digest food and constipation. SIBO was encouraged by changes in the pH of the small intestine. This led to a tryptophan, and resultant serotonin deficiency producing a subsequent increase in pain/lowering of the pain threshold, rendering her more vulnerable to offenses of other people. Cellular ATP production had come to a standstill causing the complete lack of energy. The brain fog was a result of lower ATP levels, high *Candida*, excess histamine, increased adenosine levels, and glyphosate toxicity of the liver.

Also, as result of SIBO, the increase in lactate led to higher histamine levels in the system and the asthma. The immune system responses generated by undigested gluten led to breaks in the intestinal lining and undigested proteins circulating throughout her body, which led to the systemic histamine responses, mast cell activation disease and activated adenosine receptor site-induced asthma.

Comprehension of these causes is through understanding the condition, homeopathic case taking of the symptom picture, and correct analysis indicating which remedies would address which symptoms. There are no tests in homeopathy that show you which remedies to use. Clinical practice is based on matching remedies to the symptoms of the person. Trial and error clarify homeopathic practice.

I had selected ***Conium*** as a remedy to match the overactive nervous response to seemingly 'negative' people. However, as this condition was still there upon the first follow up, I selected the more suited remedy ***Aqua amniotica*** to further repair the insult of glyphosate against the digestive lining, increase serotonin levels, and heal her perceived traumatic experience of the family she was borne into.

Natrum phosphoricum lowered histamine levels, addressed SIBO, and elevated lactate levels by reducing lactic acid. The **Glyphosate Clearing Protocol** worked to release her system from its effects.

While this is a rapid turnaround, I expect she will need continued support for following next year to maintain health and continue to repair the damages to the intestinal lining. Symptoms that have remained or relapsed are the burning in the mouth and food sensitivities, all-be-it much less. Repeating the entire protocol after a few months ought to clear this. One may ask, why wait a few months? What I understand about detox is that the body is only willing to give up so much toxin at one time. Also, based on our relation to the passing of the seasons, and daylight levels, there are times of the year when our body is more readily able to detox: spring and fall being the best times. In order to work with the seasons and the body's willingness to release it is better to rest a few months and then repeat the process rather than duplicating the sequence immediately.

Follow up a few months later confirmed my assumptions. Upon deeper case taking we discovered a history of Epstein-Barr virus and immune suppression. Accordingly, we set the course of ***Carcinosin*** and ***Glandular fever***, coupled with ***Phosphoric acid*** (due to extreme energy depletion; lack of ATP production), repeated twice, to down regulate the transactivated inflammatory response glyphosate was causing this latent RNA virus, followed by a second clearing with ***Glyphosate***.

5. **My Story of Glyphosate Toxicity**:

In 1998 I moved to the Midwest from Colorado. Previously I had lived in California. In June of 2006, after being treated with homeopathy for over 20 years I became ill with sudden onset hyperthyroidism. This came on two to three weeks after I had moved a ten-ton truckload of farm soil. For several years before I had experienced extreme mental, emotional, and physical stress which I thought contributed to this breakdown. In a matter of weeks, I was experiencing rapid heart rate, extreme weight loss, and exhaustion. That same summer in late August, I contracted whooping cough and between the two illnesses I became so weak I was sure I would die. I was bed-ridden for several weeks, too weak to talk, to walk to the bathroom, or to cook for myself. The whooping cough racked my body and depleted whatever energy stores I had left. The whooping cough took three months to resolve and slowly I regained some energy but remained to be operating at about a 3/10 energy level for the next year as the hyperthyroidism continued.

In my journey of self-healing, rather than rushing to the doctor for medication or even a diagnosis, I spent about a year in contemplative meditation examining all the factors in my life that may have contributed to the preexisting stress and possible explanation as to why I had become so sick. I was struck by how it was I that sick, especially after using homeopathy for the previous twenty-five years. How had I gotten so sick if homeopathy was a cure all medicine? Had I not been working on increasing my health and vitality all these years?

I thought the hyperthyroidism was because I lived in the Midwest away from the ocean, where there is a deficiency of iodine and selenium, both minerals necessary for healthy thyroid function. I noticed that whenever I traveled away from the Midwest and was by the ocean I felt better. And when I arrived back in the Minneapolis or Chicago airports, as soon as I was outside, the symptoms returned. Now after looking at the map of agricultural use of glyphosate in the US, I can see that it is an environmental toxin and returning home meant returning to the toxicity.

In the first years I worked with homeopathy to resolve the underlying causes in my body and psyche as best as I could. While homeopathy was working for these things, it could not touch nor modulate any of the hyperthyroid symptom expression (despite homeopathic literature full of remedies that address the thyroid). It seemed my thyroid disease was resilient to homeopathy. I thought this was odd, as homeopathy should address everything. I gave up on homeopathy as I thought it had failed me. After one year of not getting better I succumbed to taking Methimazole (the conventional medication for hyperthyroidism).

It took me ten years to recover my baseline energy and all other aspects of exhaustion and mental emotional stress, but I continued the Methimazole as the hyperthyroidism continued. During that time, I was able to reduce the Methimazole to a minimal dose, however, I could not completely get off it. Muscle testing showed I was not converting free T4 to free T3 and the glycine and heme (Fe^{+})-dependent enzymes and receptor sites in the thyroid were not functioning. Deficiency in the selenium dependent enzyme iodothyronine deiodinase led to failure to convert T4 to T3. Over time, my TSH levels had normalized but if I tried to remove the medication the rapid heart rate and weight loss would return.

The symptoms listed here are the ones that resolved during my recovery process prior to doing a **Glyphosate Clearing Protocol** and detox. The last to go were those related to the thyroid and digestive issues. My symptoms included: extreme hunger, excessive weight loss (I lost 25 pounds from 140 down to 115 in three months: I'm 5' 7"), excessive hair loss, extreme fatigue, insomnia, irritability and emotional instability, depression, and heart palpitations (115 beats per min). In addition to the weight loss, all connective tissues in my body became weak and unable to support my physical structure (collagen issues). I developed what seemed like tension headaches like my brain was squeezed in a vice, especially after drinking wine (glyphosate contamination) or when I had my menstrual cycle (iron depletion). Bloating and systemic inflammation or water retention after eating wheat products was there also. I had the beginnings of environmental sensitivity to perfumes, detergents, and artificial fragrances. At one point I developed skin lesions that looked like skin cancer on my face and legs. Chiropractic care and yoga were not holding my spine in alignment. My immune system was taxed by the whooping cough, but the susceptibility to contracting it was established by exhaustion and immune system suppression of the immune system by activation of the adenosine receptor sites, and hyperthyroidism: All conditions produced by glyphosate toxicity.

It was not until I attended a Weston A. Price Conference in the fall of 2017 when I had the opportunity to listen to Stephanie Seneff explain how glyphosate toxicity disrupts T4 to T3 conversion that it dawned on me that I had glyphosate toxicity. I recalled that just prior to the onset of the hyperthyroidism I had moved that truckload of farm soil. The farm soil must have been laden with glyphosate. I have no proof, but all logic leads to this understanding. Upon that realization I embarked on developing the process of detoxification described in this book.

One interesting thing to note is that in the year prior to the clearing protocol, I had begun making sourdough bread with Einkorn wheat. However, when starting my sourdough starter, I was confused when it was not fermenting the way the instructions had noted: that by handling the starter mix in your hands you would be imparting *Lactobacillus* bacteria which would govern the fermentation process. I thought that my starter would be rich because I had only ever taken antibiotics once 40 years ago and I always ate yogurt and natural ferments. I was wrong. Glyphosate had destroyed my biome, not only in my intestines but on my skin too. I ended up making my starter from a live probiotic supplement. This disrupted biome would explain for the bloating in my digestive track and inflammation of my intestines particularly around the ileocecal valve. This inflammation caused spasms in the connective tissues of the associated lumbar vertebrae resulting in a twist up my entire spine and pain in my liver.

I completed the **Glyphosate Clearing Protocol** described herein during the winter of 2018. Since then I was able to reduce and ween myself completely off the Methimazole and my thyroid function established normality along with the rest of my health. It is not until after the detox process was completed that I have come to understand that what I had surmised was true. If it were not glyphosate that caused the hyperthyroidism, then an ascending potency scale of the homeopathic preparation of ***Glyphosate*** would not have solved the problem. After all, isn't hyperthyroidism viewed by conventional medicine as a chronic incurable condition requiring removal or destruction of the thyroid to resolve?

In the early summer of 2018, during spraying season, some of the symptoms of glyphosate toxicity developed again, extreme fatigue, burning in my mouth, heart palpitations, bloating, and systemic inflammation. I completed a second clearing where upon all symptoms resolved.

The body detoxes in layers: the first clearing gets the bulk of the toxins out but sometime later the body starts releasing deeper stores and you need to work through the process again. Also, as glyphosate is in all conventional food products and even contaminates those products that are labeled organic which are grown in proximity to conventional crops, it would make sense that there has been continued exposure. The ground water is contaminated and, as I live in the leeward side of the farmlands of Minnesota, it is not unreasonable to deduce that I was more recently re-contaminated through air pollution from the spring spraying as well as everyone else in this state.

My Detox Experience:

I developed this protocol as I myself went through it. I had experience with cleanses as in the **Fast and Colon Cleanse**. I started the process slowly, adding the collagen and detox supplements each day, adding in the saunas and then ascending potencies of ***Glyphosate***. I cleaned out my cupboards of all conventional wheat products and anything that had glyphosate in it. A few weeks into the process, one night after a sauna had initiated a fast release of glyphosate from my tissues, my liver ceased to release bile between 11 p.m. and 3 a.m. This caused an intense paralyzing headache and needing to curl up and lay on my right side and cry. After 45 minutes of intense pain and confusion I took the remedy ***Bryonia***. Slowly my liver started to drain, and the headache decreased. Then once the glyphosate had passed to my intestines, an intense spasm and cramping caused violent intestinal pain. I was crying out in pain, which forced me to bend double, and curl onto my hands and knees. ***Colocynthis*** was indicated to release the spasm which helped to move the stool down and out.

That morning I passed the weirdest gluey, sticky, foul-smelling stool looking like plastic. At some time after this I had another dumping of glyphosate through my liver which paralyzed me with a headache again. This time I felt the intense necessity to want to kill myself. This was quite scary as I am not suicidal. I am not sure if it was the pain that was driving me or the fact that glyphosate goes so against nature that by its own essence my mind was wanting to obey its operative.

During the two months it took to cleanse my body the skin on my torso, upper thighs, chest, and back was broken out in hundreds of small, itching, and burning, non-healing skin ulcers. Saunas made things worse in the beginning as glyphosate was being liberated, then they made things better once it was clear. During this time, I was also receiving Rolfing which helped to liberate more glyphosate from my collagen and helped to integrate the collagen supplementation into my fascia. My need for the thyroid medication (methimazole) dropped off and I quickly gained weight as I was still eating the amount I was used to. Now being off the medication for some time, I do well on smaller meals and my weight has normalized. My sensitivity to artificial fragrances has remained, but I have come to learn that these are toxins too so best to avoid anyways.

During the spring of 2018, spaying season, my thyroid became hyper again, calling upon me to take the methimazole medication for several weeks. I remain sensitive to air pollution and wine contaminated with glyphosate. On those days, when I am affected, my system shuts down and I can't think straight. The burning in my tongue came back and remained for the summer. I repeated the nutritional detox and repeated the clearing potencies of ***Glyphosate*** and have remained well into the winter.

I no longer have bloating, my spine is stronger and able to hold chiropractic adjustments for longer times, and my thyroid is better. My body and mind are strong. However, I eat a very limited diet of only organic foods, only eat einkorn wheat, grass-fed beef, and organic vegetables, preferably from my garden or locally grown. I wonder what next year will bring during the spraying season?

Comments: The main remedies needed in my case during detoxification were ***Bryonia*** and ***Colocynthis*** based on the specific symptom presentation I developed during the active detox phase along with ***Glyphosate***. Prior to realizing I had been poisoned with glyphosate, yet still suffering under its effects, the main remedies I had used to sustain my health were ***Carcinosin***, ***Tuberculinum***, ***Aurum***, ***Aurum iodatum***, ***Ferrum metallicum***, ***Ferrum phosphoricum***, ***Ferrum iodatum***, ***Stannum***, ***Aqua marina***, and a few others. In retrospect I can understand why they were indicated and why they helped. ***Carcinosin*** was needed to address my energy system which in the ten years I was sick would collapse every few months. It was not until I took ***Glyphosate*** though, was I able to stop the thyroid medication. ***Tuberculinum*** is indicated in most hyperthyroid cases. ***Carcinosin*** if there is a history of EBV as well, but not in my case as I never had mono. ***Aurum***, ***Aurum iodatum***, and ***Aqua marina*** helped with the grief and despair over my loss of health and prolonged recovery, and the ramifications of an unregulated endocrine system leading to emotional instability. ***Ferrum*** and ***Ferrum iodatum*** boosted my iron levels and mainlined my health during menstruation. ***Stannum*** was a game changer for the level of exhaustion I would collapse into.

Over time I came to observe that the intestinal bloating, water retention, and inflammation around my abdomen had returned. Where upon taking the ***Polio*** nosode and observable change in digestive function occurred: stools were more formed, I no longer was retaining water, and all symptoms of distention disappeared. Polio virus enabled the tight junctions of my intestine to close. As a school-aged child I had received the oral polio vaccine. Throughout my life I have been blessed with a healthy appetite and never any food sensitives, no history of antibiotics, and intellectual discriminatory powers enabling me to choose healthy eating habits.

> **Glyphosate toxicity took me by surprise, but it has led me on a journey to discover its toxic effects and the way out of succumbing to them. It took ten years from the onset of hyperthyroidism that I become aware that glyphosate was the operator of this condition. During the first two years I took a journey within to address what might be coming from my own soul. It took 7 years to recover my strength. By doing the cleansing protocol described herein I cleared glyphosate from my body. From the compilation of research necessary for writing this book I found a solution for my body and soul. It was the direct application towards my own health of the detoxification methods described herein that saved me. In due course potentially many others will also find salvation from this work**

18. Blessings

Good luck with it all. While doing this cleanse talk to anyone and everyone you know about this poison. It will destroy all the food on the planet, all the bugs that live in the soil, all the animals that eat plants grown in this now dead soil and harm the children that are being raised on the farmland near where the toxin is being sprayed.

May we begin to rectify our actions against ourselves and call upon each other to participate in a world that is not driven by greed, fear of lack, and disconnect from nature.

May we pray that the Great Mother Earth love and bless us for the transgressions we have made against her and ourselves and help us to find reason once again. May we be free.

Amen.

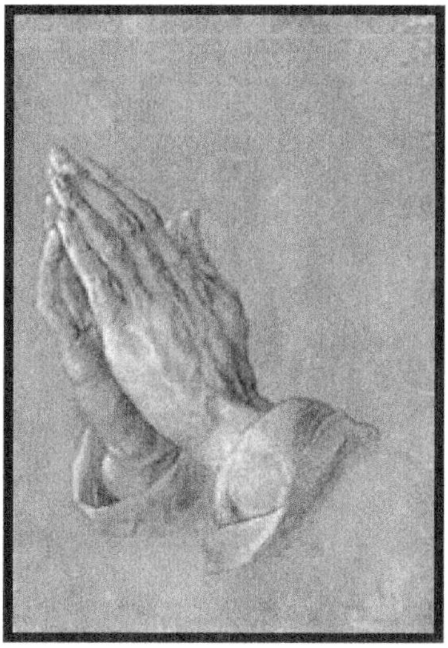

19. Fast and Colon Cleanse

Some things to think about:

Cleansing our intestines is a psychological and physiological phenomenon. It allows one to move on from the past and receive the new without debris left over to encumber us. Cleansing the upper and lower intestines stimulates the eliminative action of all cells in the body so that they can release the toxins that have been building up over the years. Before a colon cleanse there are often layers and/or pockets of debris that are deposited along the sides of the colon. These too can be there for years despite daily bowel movements.

Stool can become impacted in the minute folds of the intestinal wall. These layers inhibit the assimilation of nutrition and the eliminative processes of the cells in the colon. Without this normal process, our bodies slowly become toxic and many disease conditions arise. Increased pain, degenerative processes, and inflammatory states are common conditions from a toxic colon. The result of this can be seen psychologically as well as physically. Without properly eliminating the past we cannot fully be in the present. The nourishment we would gain from our current socio/phycological environment becomes limited. Memory becomes weak, understanding and comprehending new information is limited, and our overall view is tainted. It is as if we are mentally toxic. The scars or fragments left from the past filter our present interpretation. Cleaning the colon rids us of the past so we can move on.

The idea of fasting in this type of cleanse is not to starve oneself but rather to flush the system. It is like an oil change and radiator flush for your car. Fluids and the psyllium husks enable the flushing while the apples, veggies, maple syrup, and blue-green algae provide many calories without burdening the system.

Other things to think about:

It is best to do this kind of cleanse in the spring or the fall. It is possible to keep active all the way through the cleanse, except the last part of Phase 2 and the first part of Phase 3. During these two to three days, relaxing around the house with little or no commitments would be best. Some planning is required to fit this part into the weekend. It is recommended that if you've never done a fast and you are 30 years or older, this fast be repeated the following year. After that, a good frequency is once every five to six years to do a thorough fast, with mini fasts once a year. Too many fasts can weaken the system. Short fasts never get into the eliminative quality that a more thorough fast like this accomplishes. If unencumbered with toxins, the body can heal many ailments. Fasting will ensure a prolonged, healthy life.

You will need:

1. **Psyllium husks**: A good brand is Zand Fiber source. They are mixed with bentonite clay and a few other good herbs. Some cleansing products are loaded with many different herbs. If you are not interested in having so many medicinal herbs, it is possible to purchase psyllium husks bulk and to mix them with Bentonite clay and capsulate them yourself. You must drink 16 oz. of water each time you take the capsules.
2. **Apples**: It doesn't matter what kind but organic is best. Plan on eating 6-10 apples a day. This is for sugars, bulk, fiber, and pectin.
3. **Lemons**: Plan for 6-10 lemons a day. Lemons have many healing properties, most importantly bioflavonoids, which are antioxidants. They will enable your liver to process the toxins as your body releases them. Lemons also help pull the bile to relieve the liver.
4. **Maple Syrup**: 100% pure, for calories.
5. **Super Blue-Green Algae**: Or some other whole-food green nutritional supplement that is not in the form of vitamins, e.g.: spirulina, wheat grass, alfalfa tea or extract. My experience is that Super Blue-Green Algae is the best because it is wild, organic, and unprocessed, plus its nutritional profile is higher than any other product.
6. **Acidophilus, Bifidus**: Or any other probiotic that will replenish the natural flora of your intestines. Probiotics are essential to good health. Not only do they help us digest our food, but they synthesize vitamins, help regulate hormonal development and influxes, help normal brain development, and otherwise keep

disease producing microbes and *Candida* away. Bacteria balances can shift over the years particularly if there has been a history of illness, antibiotic use, heavy medication or alcohol consumption, which has left a system vulnerable to unhealthy bacterial populations. Dysbiosis of the bowel sometimes needs to be corrected homeopathically. Often, taking probiotics is not enough to change the condition, considering that the dysbioitic bacteria are the ones that survive in the intestines given the toxic environment. Certainly, cleansing is helping to change the environment so that healthy bacteria can begin to thrive.

7. **Other**: Fruit and vegetable juices: pear, apricot, prune, papaya, carrots, celery. Honey, molasses, rice, miso, grape seed extract, olive oil, flax seed oil, milk thistle extract, cranberry juice (100% pure), parsley tea, dandelion root, cayenne.

Tools:

- One enema bulb or bag. I found the bulb to be easier to handle.
- Loofa for scrubbing the skin.
- Discipline, courage, fortitude, and foresight.

Supplemental programs (see Appendixes):

- Retention enema.
- Gallbladder cleanse.
- Liver cleanse.
- Urinary tonic.
- Rice soup.
- Fast drink.
- Epson salt baths.
- Shiatsu massage, Swedish massage, Reflexology massage, colonic massage. (Consult your local practitioners for these services).

Program:

Phase One – Elimination

Duration 3-7 days. The duration of this part depends on several factors. The first is what kind of a diet you normally have:

- People who eat red meat every day or every other day should spend a full 7 days in this part.
- For those who eat meat seldomly and chicken or fish occasionally, 3-4 days should be good.
- Vegetarians can spend 2-3 days doing this and vegans need only 1-2 days.
- People with a fast metabolism can reduce the time while those with a slow metabolism should increase the time.

This phase is about the elimination of meat and dairy products and the introduction of a more vegetarian diet: potatoes, pasta, beans, whole grains, and fruits and vegetables. Eat lots of squash, cruciferous veggies, and dark leafy greens, 2-3 portions of vegetables/meal. Eat organic sources.

Also eliminate fried food, coffee and caffeine tea, soda pop, foods with refined flour or sugar, processed food, and alcohol.

Add to your diet:

- Apples, 4-5/day.
- 2-3 capsules of blue-green algae.
- Psyllium husks. Start with 1-2/meal, then increase the quantity each day by 1-2 per meal. Some people experience some gas from the husks. If this is the case your bowels aren't moving fast enough.
- Increase your fluid uptake, up to 3 quarts of juice, tea, and/or water.
- Massage your colon.
- Start with the coffee enemas.

Phase Two – Cleansing

Part 1) Duration 2-3 days: This phase serves to get as much bulk as possible moving through your colon and still ensure that you have enough caloric intake to sustain yourself. By this time, you should have had no meat for at least 7 days and no dairy or refined foods for 4 days. You should now eliminate complex carbohydrates and beans from your diet. You must find things that will satisfy your desires without spoiling the fast. It's better to sit down and make a meal of the following things rather than snacking all day long.

Plan 5-6 small meals each day and consume the following:

- Hot rice soup (see Appendix 2).
- Fast drink 3-4 quarts/day.
- 1-2 apples/meal.
- 3-5 psyllium husk capsules/meal.
- 2-3 algae/meal.
- Other veggies like carrots and fruit juices.

Incorporate one coffee retention enema/day, preferably in the afternoon. If you start to experience headaches, a bad taste in your mouth, or bad breath, you can be assured that now you are detoxing. Drink more fluids.

During this time, you can also add: Liver Cleanse, Gallbladder Cleanse, and Urinary Tonic (see Appendices).

Towards the end of this phase you will start to daydream about all the wonderful decadent foods you are missing. This is where the discipline, courage, fortitude, and foresight come into play. You may also start to feel a greater sense of freedom, more energy, and greater mental alertness.

Part 2) Duration 1-2 days. This is the hardest yet most rewarding part of the fast and should be planned for the weekend. During this part of the fast you will only consume:

- The fast drink: 2-3 quarts/day.
- Psyllium husks and algae: Increase up to 14 capsules/day.
- Add *acidophilus* or another probiotic.
- Continue with one enema/day.

Whereas before your stool may have been multicolored with hard lumps of matter (bits and pieces that have probably been in your intestines for several years), now it should be uniform and flaky. If you are feeling weak eat some honey or molasses straight out of the jar, or organic maple syrup. rice and barley syrups are also good.

You will know when this part of the fast is over. You may find that you are feeling pretty good and that you don't need to start eating quite yet. Take it as far as you can go. And, whereas you might have noticed that your tongue was coated white or yellow, you will now find that it is clean and there is a pleasant, sweet taste in your mouth. Any post-nasal or sinus congestion may have cleared, your skin will have cleared up, your eyes will be sparkly and clear, and your body odor may be none. If, however, this is not yet the case you need to stay in this part of the fast another day or two longer. If possible, get one or two massages during this time as they help with the elimination process.

Phase Three – Rebuilding

Duration 3-4 days. The beginning of this phase is also hard. Our inclination is to start eating a lot, but if you do, you will experience a great deal of discomfort. So, you must start slowly. It's mostly a reversal of the second and first phases:

- Eat cooked apples, fruit juices like papaya or tomato.
- Cook some more rice soup, or potato soup. Add well-cooked vegetables.
- Too many raw vegetables will be hard on the system. Make sure you avoid spicy foods, bananas (leads to constipation), and avocados (too much fat unless there are sufficient bile acids and bile salts to emulsify). In time, with eating, the liver will produce more.
- Cut back on psyllium husks and algae but continue with probiotics.
- You must wait for a good easy bowel movement before introducing more complex carbohydrates and refined foods.

After this, your body will tell you what you really want to eat, and you may find that what you thought was good before the fast now does not appeal to you. You may also find you have to eat less than you did as your ability to absorb nutrients is higher. There is also a good chance that you will see more clearly through the choices in your life and will avoid those situations that are not healthy for you. More than anything, you will have gained a profound understanding of your weaknesses and any issues about food you may have had.

Most of all you will have a renewed vitality and gusto for life.

Appendix 1) Coffee retention enema: Some say this is the best and only way to take your coffee. You may find this to be true. The idea behind this type of enema is to implant the solution and then to hold it in your bowels for 10-15 minutes. In this form, the coffee acts as an astringent so that it will help remove the crusts from inside your colon; it will also stimulate your liver and intestinal cells to eliminate. To make enough for several days boil two tablespoons of coffee in a quart of water for 10-15 minutes. You want a strong coffee. Strain the coffee and let cool to body temperature. Unused coffee can be refrigerated and heated as needed.

The easiest way to do this is to pour a bath, implant the enema, and soak in the bath for 10 minutes or so. The best way to implant the enema is to start on your hands and knees with your butt up in the air (sitting on the toilet works too). After lubricating the tip of the tube with some oil, insert it in your rectum and squeeze the bulb. Refill as needed. As you proceed with the fast you should be able to implant up to a quart of liquid at a time. Get in the bath quickly and lie down.

While you are in the bath massage your colon. Start by lying on your left side. Massage up your left side, then roll on your back. Massage across the transverse colon towards your right side, then roll onto your right side and massage down your ascending colon. Now massage the other way, ending up on your left side again. In this way you have massaged the coffee up your colon and back down. By this time, you will be ready for the toilet. It is also possible to rinse your colon with water and lemon juice after or to implant *acidophilus* by dissolving the probiotic in a fresh enema solution. During part two of **Phase Two** you want to implant probiotics in your colon to propagate a healthy biome. The lemon wash beforehand sets the pH.

Appendix 2) Gallbladder cleanse: At 11:00 pm, before bed, drink 1/4 cup olive oil with the juice of one lemon. This is to facilitate the passage of any gallstones. Do this three night in a row.

Appendix 3) Liver cleanse*:* For 3-5 days during the fast, incorporate alfalfa tea, milk thistle extract, burdock root tincture, grapefruit seed extract, and dandelion root (or any other herbs mentioned in this book). These strong bitters add nourishment and will stimulate healthy liver elimination. Aloe vera can be taken internally: 1-2 oz. a day for no more than seven days.

Appendix 4) Urinary tonic*:* As the kidneys will be called into action to filter many toxins out of the body, toning them will help support this important organ. Drink a quart of 100% pure cranberry juice diluted with water and add honey if you like. Make parsley tea by steeping chopped parsley and stinging nettles in boiled water. Drink some of this every day for 3-4 days.

Appendix 5) Rice soup: Water, garlic, onion, miso, white rice, turmeric, cumin, salt, and lime juice. Sauté onions and garlic until golden, add water, rice and spices. When rice is cooked, add miso (do not boil after adding miso), lime juice, and serve.

Appendix 6) Fast drink: 2-3 lemons, 1-2 tbsp. maple syrup, one quart of filtered water, dash of cayenne powder.

Appendix 7) Epson salts: Baths are a very important part of cleansing. They facilitate your tissues to release toxins. Use one to two cups of Epson salts per bath: W]while bathing, scrub the skin with a loofa, always towards the heart.

Appendix 8) Massage and shiatsu are vitality important to increasing circulation, cellular respiration (Krebs cycle), and opening elimination pathways. One or two massages during the cleanse is necessary.

Other books by Kate Birch

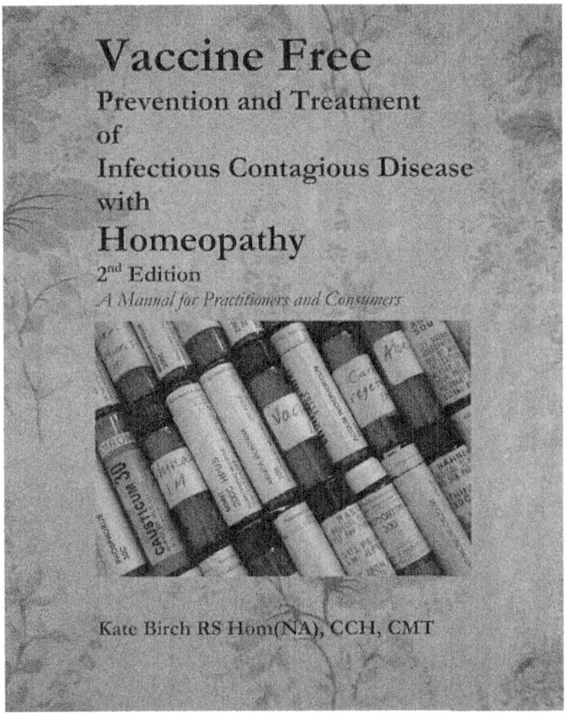

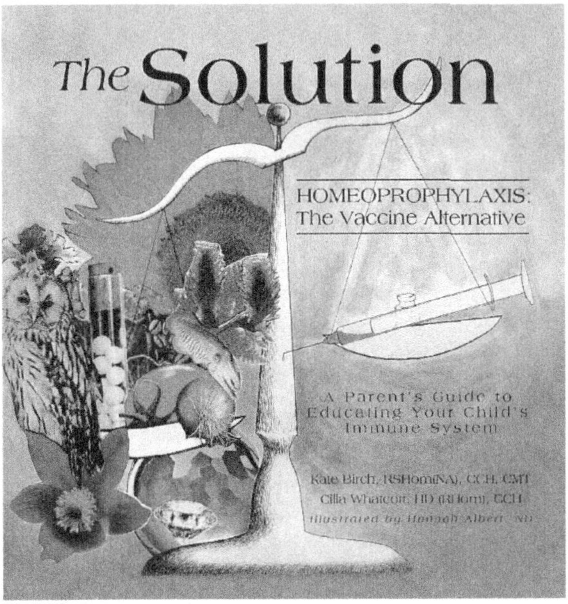

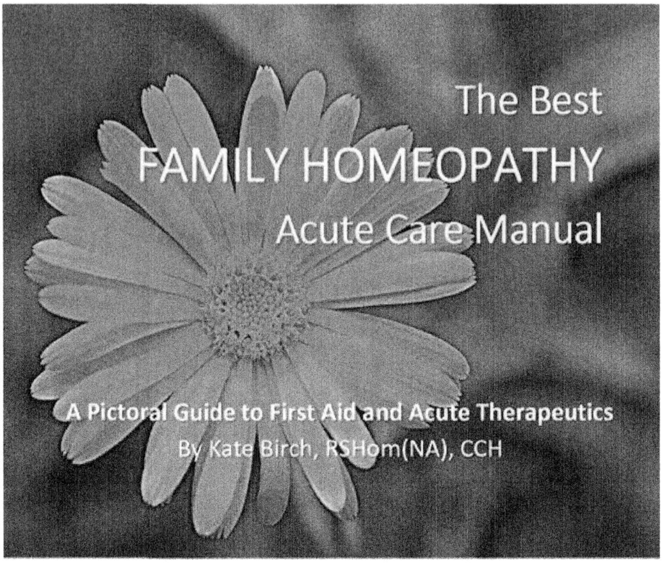
The Best
FAMILY HOMEOPATHY
Acute Care Manual
A Pictoral Guide to First Aid and Acute Therapeutics
By Kate Birch, RSHom(NA), CCH

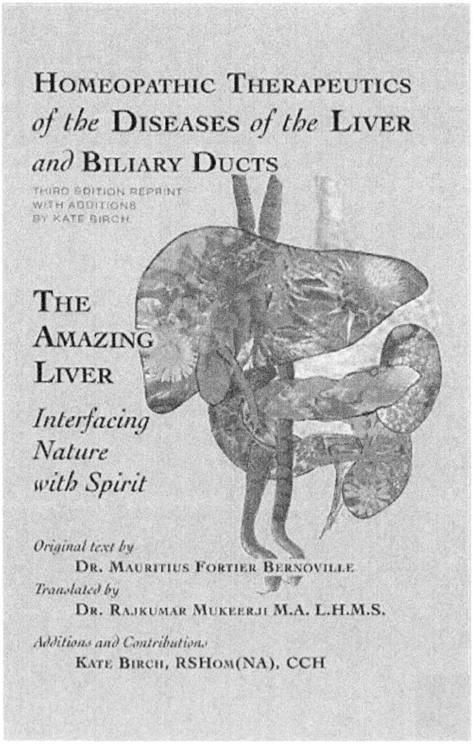
HOMEOPATHIC THERAPEUTICS
of the DISEASES of the LIVER
and BILIARY DUCTS
THIRD EDITION REPRINT
WITH ADDITIONS
BY KATE BIRCH
THE
AMAZING
LIVER
Interfacing
Nature
with Spirit
Original text by
DR. MAURITIUS FORTIER BERNOVILLE
Translated by
DR. RAJKUMAR MUKEERJI M.A. L.H.M.S.
Additions and Contributions
KATE BIRCH, RSHOM(NA), CCH

20. Index

A

B

C

D

E

F

G

H

I

J

K

L

M

N

R

S

T

U

V

W

X

Y

Z

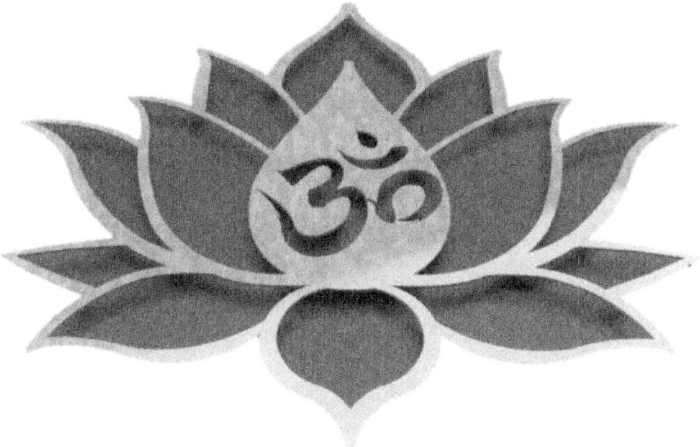

Printed in Great Britain
by Amazon

46346021R00159